Obesity is a global pandemic, which, as the Convisers emphasize, needs a new paradigm of thinking. On one hand, the book explains why our whole society has failed in the battle against obesity. On the other hand, this resource offers practical tools and approaches that are designed to help both individuals and healthcare providers to beat it. Professional, yet simple and easy to read, this book will take you through the "UnWeighted" approach, and how the correct attitude and behavior can ultimately positively affect health. I highly recommend it.

Naama Constantini, MD, DFM, FACSM, Dip. Sport Med. (CASM)
Director, Sport Medicine Center, Shaare Zedek Medical Center
Chair, National Council for Women's Health, Ministry of Health
Exercise is Medicine Center, The Hebrew University of Jerusalem

This book is brilliant because it emphasizes the patient's "why" for weight loss, not the "how much." The anti-BMI diet is one of many useful tools provided in this book. As a lifestyle medicine physician and a health and wellness coach, I have seen the power of collaborating with patients to co-create a personalized behavior change plan versus the frustration and failure of cajoling patients into the healthcare provider's weight loss plan.

Elizabeth Pegg Frates, MD
Clinical Assistant Professor, Harvard Medical School
Board of Directors, American College of Lifestyle Medicine

Overweight and obesity is a multifaceted condition that is far more complex than just achieving a proper balance between food intake and energy expenditure. Healthcare providers need to do more than just tell their patients and clients what to change—they need to help them learn how to make sustained change. This book discusses the health implications of overweight and obesity, while addressing the emotional hardships and behavioral challenges contributing to weight management struggles. It is well-written for the healthcare professional, yet easy to read.

Laura J. Kruskall, Ph.D., RDN, CSSD, LD, FACSM, FAND
Associate Professor and Director, UNLV Nutrition Sciences

As a physician specializing in sports medicine, working with professional athletes involved with collision sports, it's obvious that the size of our athletes, as well as the nation at large, is getting even bigger and bigger. In fact, the number of 300-pound athletes has quadrupled in the NFL over the last 25 years. *UnWeighted Nation* offers suggestions of where to start the dialogue and provides viable strategies and possible solutions to this serious situation, as well as the medical issues associated with obesity. This one-of-a-kind book details a new way of thinking about the problem.

Gordon W. Nuber, MD
Professor of Clinical Orthopedic Surgery, Northwestern University
Team Physician, Chicago Bears

Because obesity is a complex health issue with many causes, there are also many interrelated solutions. This major health problem can only get worse if we do not change the way we think about possible solutions and how to apply them. This book does an excellent job of discussing the various approaches that are needed by each one of us and by all levels of society.

James Skinner, Ph.D., FACSM
Past President, American College of Sports Medicine

UNWEIGHTED NATION ™
Addressing the Obesity Crisis Through Cultural Change

Jenny H. Conviser, Psy.D., CEDS, CC-AASP

Jason Conviser, Ph.D., FACSM

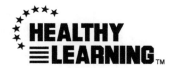

ISBN: 978-1-60679-390-9
Library of Congress Control Number: 2017939422
Book layout: Cheery Sugabo
Cover design: Cheery Sugabo

Healthy Learning
P.O. Box 1828
Monterey, CA 93942
www.healthylearning.com

DEDICATION

Since we started writing *UnWeighted Nation*, we were keenly aware of the populations whom we wanted to support. They spoke to us and us to them. Throughout the process we both listened, and we heard.

To all the professionals, including teachers, healthcare providers, counselors, and exercise specialists, who are willing to consider weight-related health with a completely new perspective and approach, we dedicate this book to you. To all the individuals who personally are challenged by weight loss, weight management, and related health matters, we dedicate this book to you. For those individuals who wish for better physical and emotional health and a viable means to do so, we dedicate this book to you. And for those individuals who support family, friends, and our nation's citizens, particularly children, on their journey to better health, we dedicate this book to you.

There is no single correct journey or end destination. We hope that this book will help you discover more of what you want, more of who you are, and more of how to achieve all that you value for your health, happiness, and well-being.

ACKNOWLEDGMENTS

We are grateful for abundant support during this writing project, without which the journey leading to its completion would not have happened. First and foremost, we thank Healthy Learning and Kristi Huelsing, publisher and managing editor, extraordinaire. Without your patience and persistence, this book would not have become a reality.

To David Goetz and Melissa Parks, we thank you for inspiring this text, launching its beginnings, and reminding us that the text and its message had considerable merit, even in those many moments when we had difficulty seeing it ourselves.

We thank all of our Ascend Consultation in Health Care staff and clients, who courageously shared their stories, and challenged our thinking as we learned daily about weight, body shape, health, and what constitutes appropriate definitions of success. We are most grateful to our friends, family and professional colleagues who reviewed chapters and inspired us to think outside the box concerning new, and sometimes controversial, approaches to weight, eating, and exercise issues.

To Becca, Sarah, and Nathan, we express our love and appreciation for sharing your energy and attention while we worked on this project, and for your editorial suggestions as we asked again and again, "how does this sound to you?"

Finally, we thank William Morgan, Ed.D., FACSM, an accomplished scientist, educator, and practitioner for his excellence in teaching and leadership. We are most grateful for his instilling an appreciation for critical evaluation, scientific rigor, and the importance of advancing current knowledge and its strategic application through vital consideration of the guiding query "what next?"

CONTENTS

PREFACE

Recently, a morning television news story was describing a product called an "Anti-Gravity Treadmill." During the narrative, it was explained that this apparatus was used to facilitate rehabilitation for lower-body injuries. This anti-gravity treadmill reportedly lifts the body and lightens the weight-bearing impact on legs and joints, as the patient exercises or rehabilitates an injury. The reduced gravitational force on the body permits progressive loading for a wide spectrum of patients with various injuries. Less weight-loading on the lower body helps the patient walk, run, jump, or climb with correct biomechanical form, while reducing pain and concurrently facilitating recovery.

Patients who used the anti-gravity device, while exercising, described the experience as "freeing." The experience helped them feel stronger, more confident, and more hopeful about their current activity, rehabilitation efforts, and potential for more progress. Physical movements that were previously more difficult now felt less so. The anti-gravity rehabilitative environment was referred to as *"UnWeighted."*

Similarly, a pressing need exists for an *"UnWeighted"* approach to better understand and address the plethora of weight-related matters that burden this nation and its people. In reality, the social, economic, medical, and financial costs of this situation, particularly obesity, are at an all-time high and continue to rise.

Despite the enormity of the problem, efforts to solve it have consistently been unsuccessful. While the underlying intent of most of these efforts has often been commendable, the wished for results simply have not been achieved. More often than not, individuals weigh more than they want or is good for their health.

Equally troubling is the fact that the various strategies and steps purported to help ameliorate weight-related issues have only served to exacerbate the circumstances confronting individuals who have a problem with their weight. The obvious and most immediate concern is identifying and implementing a feasible course of action that can help these individuals—one that is both viable and results-oriented.

UnWeighted Nation: Addressing the Obesity Crisis Through Cultural Change offers a practical and logical model for dealing with weight-related matters, one that is grounded in cultural change… one that actually works. Unlike the traditional array of efforts to affect change in a person's weight, which collectively tend to have a singular focus on the numerics (e.g., lose this much weight in this much time, eat this much food on this particular schedule; etc.). The *"UnWeighted"* model advocated in this text steps away from the numerics. It then details how to effectively alter the factors that have contributed to the individual's situation.

UnWeighted Nation: Addressing the Obesity Crisis Through Cultural Change is designed to transform feelings of futility and hopelessness to a sense of confident optimism.

Jenny Conviser

Jason Conviser

The Challenge

If shame were as measurable as weight, hers was off the charts. She did not need a scale or a healthcare provider to remind her. She recalled daily her attempts at in vitro fertilization and being told her weight was the reason she still wasn't pregnant. Defeated, she signed up again for a meal replacement plan. Maybe "this time," she would keep off the weight.

He felt punished for being overweight. In the fall of his sophomore year, he trailed behind his classmates in the one-mile run, walking more than he ran. While he completed the course, his time—combined with his other sub-par scores on the various President's Council on Physical Fitness test measures—landed him in the lower-fit gym class. Labeled by his peers as "fat gym," his physical education class was a grueling hour of drills and calisthenics. On the other side of the gym, the "not-fat" gym class happily played volleyball.

She was dying. At least, it felt like that. Her chest tightened with each wheeze and gasp for breath. "Let's go to the doctor," her husband urged, recognizing this possible asthma attack was worse than the last. She refused. Having regained the 80 pounds she lost the previous summer, as well as putting on an additional 10 pounds, she feared the scale and the ensuing doctor's reprimand more than suffocation.

After 25 years employment with the same airline, she agreed to relocate. The cross-country trek promised a move up the corporate ladder. Just a year later, management pulled her aside and informed her that she didn't fit the corporate image. They had to let her go, even though she had contributed to the successful operations of the business. While not explicit, the message was that her weight was a liability.

A Fortune 500 executive was a rock star in the boardroom, negotiating multi-million-dollar deals, but he was afraid of walking down the street. If he fell, how would he get up?

Fearing the anticipated scrutiny and judgment that inevitably accompanies summer's cropped tops and blue jean shorts, she started the "Kale Diet." Kale would be all she consumed for days. She has episodes of feeling intense hunger, dizzy, light-headed, and weak, and has difficulty focusing on her work. Unexpectedly, seeing a freshly baked and frosted cake on the counter at home, she has one piece, then two, and then more. A lot more. Until she feels ill. While she experiences relief in being refueled, she also feels desperation, fueled by her fear for consequences for her body that she has worked so hard to sculpt. Panicked, she runs to the bathroom to throw up.

She has wonderful friends, graduated from an enviable higher institution, is beautiful, smart, competitive, athletic, fit, and of healthy weight. She is on top of the world as a young professional, when she is unexpectedly diagnosed with an aggressive and difficult to treat deadly illness. Her team of top doctors create a plan of treatment and lay out the details for her and her parents. Near the end of this meeting, feeling scared and overwhelmed, she asks her doctors if there is anything she can do to help herself. They suggest a "low-fat diet." She jumps in and commits to a low-fat diet. Subsequently, thinking that meat has some fat, she eliminates meat from her diet entirely and eventually finds her way to the "no-fat" and almost the "no-food" plan. Her weight plummets; her appetite disappears; she becomes fearful of eating. As a result, she loses 40 percent of her body weight in the next several months. While the illness did not threaten her life, the food, body-related obsessions and weight loss almost killed her.

The first-grade teacher was the boy's biggest supporter, developing a "two thumbs up" code to signal when his pants were falling down. Too many times, the boy was taunted: "Hey, fatty, your butt is hanging out!" But the reality was, she couldn't save him. Living in a tsunami zone, the school regularly practiced up-hill evacuation drills that the obese child could barely complete. In the event of a real tsunami, the teacher was told to "leave the child behind."

Friends and family younger and older gathered to celebrate the new wedding engagement. Everyone was excited to hear the news. Who was this new lucky guy newly engaged to this gorgeous, bright and lovely young lady? After learning some details about the new "fiancé," a twenty something year old friend asked the "bride to be" a question, "So what are you doing for your wedding?" The older members of the gathering had falsely assumed that the question referenced details like wedding location, honey moon plans and flower colors, etc. Wrong. The question actually targeted the bride's choice of "weight loss plan."

An accomplished, academy award winning actress arrives up for the first reading of the new script. She is beyond talented and exquisitely beautiful. After the reading, the producer approaches her and asks if she can just "lose five pounds."

Every family, every community, and every corporate environment hosts millions of stories of people affected by weight or obesity-related matters—lives often weighted down by defeat, fear, shame, stigma, and debilitating health. Over the last 30 years, obesity has become a national epidemic, with repercussions not only for the person struggling with their weight but for the entire nation.

The *American Journal of Public Health* reported that 18 percent of deaths among Americans ages 40 to 85 are related to obesity. Original estimates had the rate at 5 percent, almost four times lower than reality. The economic consequences are breathtaking. Some estimates indicate that by 2018, healthcare costs related to obesity in the U.S. will exceed $300 billion per year. By 2030, lost productivity caused by obesity will cost the nation more than $500 billion dollars annually. Arguably, worsening rates of childhood obesity may be contributing to the rise in rates of obesity among adults. Experts report that childhood obesity rates have tripled in the past 30 years. In fact, 12.5 million children and teens are obese, with obesity rates increasing across the age span, diverse ethnic groups and socio-cultural groups. Research indicated that more than 30 percent of children between ages 2 and 19 had a BMI (body mass index) at or above the 85th percentile for their age.

Obesity that begins in childhood tends to persist into adulthood. Many children do not simply "grow out of it," as they would a pair of sneakers. Once obese, neurochemical, biological, and triggered genetics further perpetuate obese conditions. Eating and exercise patterns might not be sufficient to counter the trend. Some experts believe that by 2030, approximately half of American adults will be obese. If ignored, this situation will devastate individuals, families, communities, healthcare institutions, and economies.

Similar to the United States, Mexico and China are also seeing a rapid escalation in rates of obesity. One in five children in China are obese. In China, 260 million adults are overweight or obese, 92 million adults are diabetic, and 177 million adults have hypertension.

In October 2011, the United Nations and the World Health Organization issued a joint communiqué that reported obesity as the single biggest healthcare concern facing the world. Professor Philip James, chairman of the International Obesity Task Force, stated, "We now know that the biggest global health burden for the world is dietary in origin and is compounded by association with low physical activity levels. This is going to plague us for the next 30 years."

What will truly plague us is obesity's collateral damage. According to the Centers for Disease Control and Prevention, obese children tend toward type 2 diabetes, metabolic syndrome, high cholesterol and high blood pressure, and asthma, as well as other breathing problems, sleep disorders, early puberty, and menstruation. In addition, emotional damage including low self-esteem, anxiety, depression, low motivation, and life-threatening eating disorders are all associated risk. Diseases that appeared in older adults, both physical and mental are now manifesting much earlier—even during adolescence. Given the weight trajectory of our children, and medicine's ability to prolong life, imagine the quality of life in their later years. Advances in medicine will keep the next generation alive longer, they just won't be healthy. Chances are they won't be happy either.

THE WAR ON OBESITY

When the enemy is clearly identified, America rallies to attack and protect its people. When the first American in Texas died of an Ebola infection in Texas, President Barack Obama nominated an "Ebola czar" to oversee this health threat, patients were transported to the Centers for Disease Control and Prevention and the National Institutes of Health, and nationwide plans were initiated to improve infectious disease care. Efforts were also undertaken to dramatically increase the number of specialized treatment centers, as well as to improve the production and availability of new medications to treat this deadly virus.

In contrast, in terms of the obesity epidemic, the government's response has been less comprehensive and less organized than its reaction to the risk of Ebola infection. For example, one government office works to increase availability of subsidized cheese and dairy products (often higher in fat content), while another office works to advertise the benefits of eating lower-fat foodstuffs. Some government officials propose taxing sugary drinks, while others indicate that this strategy is ineffective in deterring consumption.

Equally inexplicable, while some government bureaucrats proclaim their recognition of the importance of exercise in helping children manage good health, the government continues to reduce the level of available funds allocated for physical education classes in schools. Furthermore, the United States Department of Agriculture (USDA) promotes dietary guidelines, while the chair of the Harvard University School of Public Health argues that such nutritional advice (i.e., a low-fat diet) is unsound and may actually contribute to rising rates of obesity. An extensive array of dietary products, remedies, and programs literally flood the market, targeted at an unsuspecting segment of the population, seeking a quick-fix to their situation. Pushing back against this state of affairs are professionals with expertise in eating disorders who warn of the hazards of buying into the empty promises of gimmicks and dietary fads. At times, it seems that Americans are at war with themselves.

While medical personnel, researchers, educators, and policymakers debate possible remedies, more and more children and adults suffer harassment, bullying, self-loathing, and isolation, as well as waning physical and emotional health. As obese children become obese adults, they likely will experience discrimination and the associated economic consequences of lower wages and a curtailed opportunity for hiring and promotion.7 Furthermore, those individuals who are not obese fear that they will become so.

The current cultural conditions can lead to unintended consequences. For example, parents of a "20-something" adult daughter, suffering life-threatening anorexia, apologized for routinely putting her on a treadmill at age four, forbidding her to eat dessert on weekdays, and lecturing her about "fat." They had been bullied and teased about weight as children, had watched their parents die prematurely due to cardiovascular disease and diabetes, and had struggled to control their own weight. In reality, they were loving, well-educated individuals who only wanted to spare their children the physical and mental anguish that they had known.

Culture has armed Americans with quick-fix diets, fat-free foods, artificial sweeteners, pills, teas, and herbal remedies—each promising to shed the pounds, and even bariatric surgery. In fact, weight loss is a multi-billion-dollar industry. It's big business. Americans are sampling everything from the paleo diets for weight loss, to protein shakes promising muscle development. Furthermore, advertisers and products often encourage children to lose weight. Body mass index and body weight are posted on report cards of children in an attempt to motivate weight loss. Yes, the problem seems obvious enough to many (it's "fat people"), and the solutions are legion. Ban cupcakes for birthday celebrations in elementary schools. Inspect children's school lunches for contraband (e.g., potato chips and cookies). Post the caloric content of foodstuffs on menus in fast food chains and restaurants. Revise the design of nutritional labels on packaged food items to improve readability, ad infinitum.

The effort to address the obesity crisis also extends to institutional elements. In 2012, for example, New York City attempted to ban sales of super-sized soda within its city limits. In Chicago, Mayor Rahm Emanuel, with the support of several major corporations, including PepsiCo and Coca-Cola, announced a weight-loss competition among 38,000 city employees and spouses of the "Windy City" and their counterparts in San Antonio, Texas. In yet another example, in 2005, Liberty University, in Lynchburg, Virginia, required overweight university students to take an extra fitness class in order to meet the requirements of graduation. While the American Beverage Association CEO, Susan Neely, reminds us that "discriminatory taxes don't change behavior," politicians move to add taxes to sugar. In a political setting, White House physician Dr. Eleanor Mariano called out New Jersey's Governor Chris Christy via CNN to "take responsibility" and lose weight.

In fact, there are more Americans on diets than ever before. Eighty-five percent of dieters are women. There are also more men dieting and more kids dieting at younger ages. In 2015, more than half of the adult individuals in America attempted to lose weight, exercising away calories, counting calories, skipping meals, popping pills, or undergoing surgery. Even television dials up the weight loss noise with the popular show "The Biggest Loser." The show appeals to Americans' deep belief that winning is getting thin fast—at any cost. Unfortunately, too many Americans are oblivious to the reality behind the "reality show": Any person who moves away from their family and work responsibilities, exercises six to seven hours a day, and is served low-energy food will lose weight. That's the truth.

The underreported story, however, according to blogs by past contestants, presents a different picture. During the show, contestants may be yelled at, called names, informed that they are not working hard enough, and accused of being weak or lazy. On occasion, they are told, "they just don't want it badly enough," as if "wanting it" means body fat reduction. Blogs also described contestants commonly abstaining from eating solid food, using colonics, sitting in saunas, spitting saliva into cups, and using other dehydrating methods to reduce weight in preparation for final weigh-ins. Ambulances and paramedics have taken away contestants who became ill or passed out. Some contestants reported peeing blood in their final weight loss weeks.

It is common knowledge, however, that any weight loss can be challenging to sustain. In the two weeks "following" the last day on the show, some contestants regain more than 30 pounds. A few individuals return to a new lifetime high weight within one year of appearing on the show. In fact, the whole story is seldom reported. Long-term data, however, indicates that rapid weight regain, medical complications, and a plethora of psychosocial difficulties can follow large and rapid weight loss.

No, Americans are not short on weight loss products or strategies. As the diet culture flourishes, so do diet product sales. Over the past 23 years, the diet market jumped from $32 billion to $62 billion.

Yet, rates of obesity worsen, and the desire for thin continues to escalate. Some brides, in an effort to lose weight prior to their wedding, have nasogastric tubes surgically inserted. A more recent weight loss aid is the "AspireAsist," a surgically implanted device that permits some ingested contents to be drained from the stomach.

Public interest seems more focused on pounds lost than on the medical or psychosocial risk. Weight loss is no longer just about health. Thin obsession has become a slippery slope, leading to frustration and fluctuating weight, as well as, on occasion, broken confidence, illness, isolation, decreased level of mood, increased risk of eating disorders, and suicide for both boys, girls, men, and women.

Matt Ryd, a young Chicago musician, took his life after a "long and tough battle with anxiety, depression, and an eating disorder." A year before his death, he posted a touching video on his struggle with his eating disorder. An intelligent, talented, handsome, and yes, slender Ryd admitted in the viral video, "Sometimes, I look in the mirror and am repulsed by what I see. I obsess over what and how much I eat. Sometimes, I've overeaten and then forced myself to throw up." The tragic end to his public journey confirms the limits of the weight loss industry and its thin ideal.

A SIZE-MATTERS WORLD

Americans live in a size-matters world. American culture demands that kids be thin, falsely believing that thin is healthy, beautiful, success, and power. For seven-year-olds and 40-year-olds alike, thin is even considered sexy cool.

A few brands, like Abercrombie & Fitch, refuse to stock women's clothing in XL or XXL sizes (nothing beyond a size 10). These corporate entities eschew overweight teens advertising their brand. "In every school, there are the cool and popular kids, and then there are the not-so-cool kids," states Mike Jeffries, CEO of Abercrombie & Fitch. "Candidly, we go after the cool kids." And his most honest line: "I don't want our core customers to see people who aren't as hot as them wearing our clothes." Honesty aside, in 2014, Jeffries was fired (despite a public apology the year before) by the company's board of directors for allegedly destroying the reputation of the business.

Other companies, like Lululemon Athletica, a "yoga-inspired" athletic apparel company, similarly positions its brand: "Our product and design strategy is built around creating products for our target guest in our size range of 2 to 12." Lululemon's positioning seems a kinder and gentler version of Abercrombie & Fitch's.

Edging out the average woman is a trend among the fashion industry. Only 10 years ago, plus-sized models averaged between size 12 and 18. Today, the majority of plus-sized models on agency rosters are between size 6 and 14, while the average woman is a size 14.

The harsh truth is that the friends of our nation's obese children are adopting Madison Avenue's biases toward overweight youth. One study of preschool girls (ages three to five) looked at how these young children internalized the "thin ideal" and attributed stereotypes to others, based on weight. The girls were asked to choose from several different game pieces, like those in the board game "Candy Land." Each piece was identical to the others in the set, except for weight. The kids chose pieces that represented themselves and a best friend.

Previous research showed that kids tended not to distinguish that much between thin and average weights. In this study, however, the girls more often chose game pieces depicting "thin" over game pieces showing the average-sized images. Their response may be associated with the trend of greater exposure of young children to the "thin ideal" through products, messaging, images, and entertainment.

America's corporate world has learned that "skinny" sells. In turn, children are learning early and repeatedly that "fat is bad." In fact, cultural awareness of the value assigned to "thin" continues to increase. The more obese our children become, the more likely they will be ostracized because of their weight—by peers, by parents, by teachers, by fitness professionals, and even by healthcare providers.

BULLYING CULTURE

It's one thing to be overweight and lonely. It's another to be overweight and hated for it, and even bullied for it. Weight bias exists in media, employment, education, healthcare, and interpersonal relationships for children, teens, and adults. "Fat hatred has become so pervasive," states Dr. Robyn Silverman, author of Good Girls Don't Get Fat: How Weight Obsession Is Messing Up Our Girls and How We Can Help Them Thrive Despite It, "that it is part of the fabric of our language and interactions." Those communications may be intended or unintended, verbal or non-verbal.

Regardless, fat hatred can translate into bullying. What makes weight-related bullying so pernicious is its subtlety. It's not physical. There are no physical blows. The bullying may simply be an innuendo at the middle-school lunch table: "Did you want my mac-and-cheese, too?" It can also be direct and deliberate, for example, "Let's Not Talk to Fat People Day."

Fat is ugly. Fat is lazy. "Fat and thin are no longer simply assessments of size or weight," says journalist Katia Hetter, "but rather of character." Overweight and obese children live in a class society, where thin tends to represent the upper class, and fat signifies a lower class characterized by their peers as ugly, stupid, lazy, and even selfish.

"Fattertainment" only adds to the stereotype and inevitable exclusion of obese youth. "Winners" on screen are frequently portrayed by thin characters, such as Mary Poppins, Snow White, and Belle. Villains are played by the chubby or obese, such as Ursula. Americans seem to love fat humor. With over three quarters of television and videos stigmatizing overweight youth, there's no shortage of opportunity. Obese characters overindulge in junk food. They rarely fall in love. Overweight cartoon characters are typically depicted as unattractive, unintelligent, unhappy, and even cruel. Harry Potter's cousin, Dudley, is portrayed as mentally slow, greedy, and fat. Dudley is the guy we laugh at and not the one from whom we expect much.

Chelsea Heuer, research associate at the Rudd Center for Food Policy and Obesity at Yale University, writes that "Research shows that grade-school children learn to make fun of overweight peers from watching television and playing video games." A recent study of 30 episodes of children's television programming, showed 66 occurrences of weight stigmatizing or disparaging images relating to size or weight. As such, fattertainment may be grooming the next generation of playground bullies. It may also be leading to a future in which that one in 20 females will suffer from an eating disorder in their lifetime.

This situation all poses an enormous challenge for parents. How do you help your child with the social rejection related to size, shape, or weight? Middle school is hard enough. What do you say to your son who walks home alone each day, while his "friends," since grade school, horse around on the other side of the street? Few teenagers might admit they intentionally avoid hanging out with overweight students, but the proof is not in what they say, but in what they do. In the face of so much negativity, how do you help your children remain thoughtful and respectful of children of all sizes?

Overweight teenagers report that they are pinged by trusted adults, including parents. Parents may be well-intending, but bribing children to lose weight with money, clothes, and opportunities appears only to make them feel insufficient, lacking, or just overall "bad." The "help" feels more like the condemnation and harassment the child experiences at school. It may not look like peer harassment, but to the child, it is just as painful or even worse, because it is coming from the people who are supposed to love and accept them most at any size.

In *The New York Times*, Harriet Brown cites a study in the journal *Pediatrics* that questioned 350 teenagers at two separate weight-loss camps. A stunning 37 percent of the respondents indicated that they had experienced what only can be called bullying from their parents. Furthermore, 42 percent of the teenagers in the study said that they had felt bullied from coaches and gym teachers. *The New York Times* article quotes one of the study's authors, Rebecca Puhl, director of research at Yale University's Rudd Center for Food Policy and Obesity: "What we see most often from parents is teasing in the form of verbal comments."

Even well-intentioned neighbors are ganging up on overweight youth and their "enabling" parents. *The Atlantic* reported that a North Dakota woman would be doling out letters instead of treats on Halloween. "Your child is, in my opinion," she writes in the letter, "moderately obese and should not be consuming sugar and treats to the extent of some children this Halloween season. My hope is that you will step up as a parent and ration candy this Halloween and not allow your child to continue these unhealthy eating habits." The "step up as a parent" message is central to many anti-obesity campaigns disseminated across America. One anti-obesity campaign, launched in Georgia, by the Children's Healthcare of Atlanta Strong4Life, was heavily critiqued for its blame and shame tactics. In one ad, a picture of a sad overweight boy is underscored with the message, "Warning: Fat prevention begins at home. And the buffet line." Another ad from the same campaign heaps more shame on the parents: "Chubby kids may not outlive their parents." Even though this strategy has been proven to be less motivating than ads that promote specific health choices and that empower parents, the shaming continues.

As the level of obesity has risen, a bullying culture that belittles people and cripples their sense of self has flourished. It is no surprise, then, that overweight kids are more likely to be depressed, bullied, and victims of violence. They have low self-esteem. These factors, individually or combined, threaten the well-being of our children, families and communities.

QUICK AND EASY

Obesity would be much easier to address if it were only about "calories in and calories out." Weight management issues would be a snap, if it were, truly, just food and exercise. It's not. It's about behavior; it's about relationships; it's about environment; it's about genetics; and much more. Some factors we can control, and many we can't.

Perhaps that's why parents, educators, healthcare professionals, mental healthcare professionals, and dieticians are frustrated. Much of what they are doing to address obesity does not always work the way we might hope. It's like a game of tug-of-war. The game demands you pull back hard to win. When you're pulling back, however, your opposition pulls in the opposite direction. Professionals and parents can force weight loss, but *results, we have learned, often, are not positive or lasting.* Obesity is a highly refractory condition. Human nature pushes back.

What adds to the complexity is how different managing weight or changing eating behaviors is from other behavioral-related changes, such as quitting smoking. If a person stops smoking, their health improves. But, people can't stop eating. Food is necessary to sustain life.

In the U.S., overweight conditions are often falsely associated with a lack of willpower, poor self-control, and a lack of nutritional knowledge. Yes, everyone could use more willpower, but the perception that obesity could be solved with a simple "yes" to more exercise and a "no" to fat and sugar is philistine. If children and adults simply needed more rules and monitoring, "parenting" or "coaching" weight would be a breeze. It's not. Furthermore, doctors would see their patients shed weight, keep it off, and report a satisfied life. They don't.

Nothing about solving the obesity epidemic is a snap. The solution is not a "fix." Amelioration will not come from unilateral intervention. The solution is not merely healthy snacks and more laps around the track. Pop culture craves the quick, the simple, and the finite. Packaged sound bites promise the same fix for everyone. While the "Let's get Americans moving" public service announcements by celebrities and politicians are laudable, arguably, they are insufficient.

However, great opportunity exists. If we allow ourselves to learn more and look more precisely, we see that the obese condition is a state of being that evolves distinctively for each individual. Obesity is the outward representation of an amalgam of conditions, varying circumstances, history, genetics, psychosocial health, biology, and environment. Each obese condition is a unique condition that can fluctuate throughout a person's lifetime. Defaulting to the formulaic is the seemingly quick and easy strategy for many. While it is tempting, we know enough about weight and physiology to know that our quick-fix interventions are not working well and may even be hazardous to an individual's health.

America's diet mentality is just one of the many outgrowths of our quick-fix culture. While it has created billions for national brands, it has not led to positive, long-term outcomes for our children. In fact, exposing children or teens early in their life to weight loss and dieting regimens may put them at risk for eating disorders.

A University of Minnesota researcher conducted a controlled study of adolescent girls in different treatment groups. The investigation found that five to seven years later, the girls with the most focus on diet, weight loss, calorie reduction, and exercise not only gained weight, they were also at a higher risk for eating disorders. Furthermore, the earlier someone is exposed to dieting, the greater the likelihood that the person will be obese, as well as the greater the degree of his or her obese condition in adulthood.

As such, the diet mentality, like so many other quick fixes for weight loss (e.g., stomach stapling, gastric bypass, liposuction, and pills, to name a few), may cause more problems than it prevents or solves. Evidence shows that dieting for many individuals leads to more problematic eating, loss of control, and weight escalation.

There certainly is no quick fix to changing the environments that contribute to obesity. Take, for instance, the dramatic rise of sedentary behaviors involving "screen-time," including television, computer, movies, YouTube, Facebook, and Facetime, among children. One study revealed that every day, American children spend seven and a half hours using some form of electronic technology with teens engaged in telephone-related activities, averaging three hours daily. Increasingly, kids are also online to confirm homework assignments, check grades, complete homework, and take tests for school. The use of this technology adds to the number of sedentary minutes in a child's day and is expected to increase over time.

It is estimated that 1.79 billion dollars are spent on food marketing for youth in the United States, with television being the primary medium to reach youth. On average, children and teens view more than 10 food-related advertisements daily or nearly 4,000 per year. As a result, by the time children have finished high school, they have viewed an estimated 87,000 fast-food commercials, states, Kelly Brownell, Ph.D.

Food availability can affect health and obesity. "Food deserts," in particular, can be a complicating factor. The President's Council on Fitness, Sports & Nutrition reports that more than 23 million Americans, including 6.5 million children, live in food deserts—areas that are more than a mile away from a supermarket. In addition, nearly 15 percent of American households cannot afford adequate food to meet their nutritional needs. Cultural, physiological, environmental, relational, and socio-economic factors converge to create a complex problem that is not easily corrected by popping a pill or prescribing a diet.

We all love simple solutions. The quick-fix approach is attractive. You have a problem. The problem is fat. The fix is no fat. Because fat is often visible, it is easy to identify as the target of intervention. Other factors, however, also have an impact on creating and sustaining the obese condition, including genetics, metabolism, affinity for exercise, lifestyle, access to exercise facilities, economics, hormone and chemical regulators of appetite and satiety, and even emotional states.

Emotion may play an important role in this regard. Emotions can influence factors like appetite, satiety, interest in food, degree of pleasure from food, ability to taste food, and much more. The nature of your relationship with yourself and your emotions, as well as your relationships with other individuals can powerfully influence your interest in certain foods, your thoughts about food, and how you consume food. Even parental emotional states can influence food and eating patterns in their children. Clearly any number of factors can influence "body size"; no one solution will stem the tide of escalating obesity in this country.

In the private sector, fewer efforts have been made to contain the floodwaters of obesity. After all, the food industry, built on the low-cost production of junk food and seemingly manufactured and processed foods that foster the addictions of humans to these foods, stands to lose billions of dollars of market share. Recently, the food industry, led by brand juggernauts like Burger King, General Foods, and the Coca-Cola Company, appeared to be laying sandbags when it launched the Children's Food and Beverage Advertising initiative, designed to encourage marketing of healthier dietary choices and a healthy lifestyle to children under 12. But not much has changed.

In fact, it might even be worse. In an article that appeared in the journal PLOS Medicine, "Thinking Forward: The Quicksand of Appeasing the Food Industry," internationally renowned expert at eating Kelly Brownell writes that "objective reports … have shown a tidal wave of marketing of calorie-dense, nutrient-poor foods to children, and if any change is occurring, marketing is on the increase." To become a partner in the battle against obesity, the implicit demand of the food industry is to sell less of their more profitable food. It seems such a demand would come at high cost.

Recently, Coca-Cola launched an obesity-awareness campaign, but the irony was too obvious not to pan. In this instance, a global brand was trying to apologize for how it makes money. Does Coca-Cola move out of the bottling and distribution business—

not at all. For the past few years, Coke has been acquiring various brands of beverages from water to juices to even coconut beverages in anticipation of a significant drop in soda consumption. Its diversification of its product line may serve as a presumptive strategy given that when it is challenged by the government and medical communities regarding its array of products, it can counter that it offers a spectrum of choices for the consumer.

Seven percent of calories of our collective diet come from soda, notes Mark Bittman, writer on food for *the New York Times* and author of the VB6 and The VB6 Cookbook. So, it's up to us to remember that Coke makes its money selling sugar-sweetened beverages," he said, "and even when they're apologizing for that, as they appear to be doing here—they're still selling them."

It's not that Coca-Cola is apologizing for their products and tremendous acumen at the distribution of its beverages all over the world. Rather, it's that it sees the current trend and has been preparing for the future where it can maintain its competitive advantage of bottling and product distribution to all parts of the globe. Its new strategy will allow consumers to make the choice that is best for them.

WEIGHT BIAS AMONG HEALTHCARE PROVIDERS

Unfortunately, the weight-related cultural values and perspectives have seeped into the doctor's office. In a study of medical students, some respondents reported that derogatory humor about obese patients was acceptable. When asked about cancer, however, students said that patients with cancer were "off limits" as targets for humor. Subsequently, one of the interviewers in the study asked a student, "So cancer trumps everything else? What if there was a morbidly obese cancer patient?" The medical student then replied, "We would still make fun of them for being obese."

Patients of all sizes may sense the dismissal, the discounting, and the disrespect. Overweight patients perceive (often correctly) that they will not be taken seriously. When a 6'0", 342-lb, 48-year-old male arrived for a scheduled office visit with his internist, complaining of pain in his left knee when walking, the physician immediately recommended fewer donuts and bariatric surgery—without examining the knee or ordering a test. Stunned, the patient couldn't wait to leave. He surmised, "I felt totally dismissed." The patient requested his records and left the office and practice. His next physician examined the man's knee, ordered tests, and diagnosed a torn meniscus.

A study of attitudes among healthcare providers confirms the biases within their profession. "Providers view patients who are obese as non-compliant, lazy, lacking in self-control, awkward, weak-willed, sloppy, unsuccessful, unintelligent, and dishonest." On occasion, obese individuals may believe that people don't like them. In many cases, they are right. Even doctors roll their eyes when they walk into the office.

The obese commonly experience disapproval and disappointment. We've discovered that those individuals who are struggling with overweight issues may have lower confidence, lower mood, and lower performance in school or work pursuits. Some may feel shame and are self-conscious. Isolation is common. The results of one study in which a "quality of life questionnaire" that was administered found that the morbidly obese with binge eating disorder, on average, report a lower quality of life and greater functional impairment than individuals in treatment for other kinds of eating disorders, mental illness, and/or addictions.

ARE AMERICANS READY?

Redefining success as something different than sustaining the stereotypically extreme, thin, frame is a cultural shift for which many individuals are not ready. Most people can't remember when they first believed that "fat" was bad. All too often, the message has been ever-present and pervasive. From "Barbies" to comic book heroes, individuals have learned to fear flab more than death.

Recently, a self-professed "plus-size" teen, Jewel Moore, started a petition, requesting Disney to produce positive plus-size protagonists—someone as "bright, amazing, and memorable as their others." A month later, Moore argued her case on the "Today" show, during which the following response from Disney was read: "There are many types of princesses, just as there are many types of girls, who each have their own unique history, character, and story. We appreciate and celebrate all types of women and girls and their own individual beauty." The movie Brave broke the princess mold, when it featured a heroine with red hair. Time will tell is appreciation of "individual beauty" will apply to a shape other than thin. Culture may not be ready for such a shift.

On occasion, a celebrity will take an anti-diet stance, like Jennifer Lawrence did during her climb to stardom. She stated, "In Hollywood, I'm obese. I'm considered a fat actress. I eat like a caveman. I'll be the only actress who doesn't have anorexia rumors! I'm never going to starve myself for a part … I don't little girls to be like, 'Oh, I want to look like Katniss, so I'm going to skip dinner!'"

In Lawrence's case, her diet defiance did not have a negative impact on her popularity. In fact, the opposite is true. An Academy Award and Golden Globe later, she is America's newest sweetheart, even earning a spot on Time magazine's 100 Most Influential list. Lawrence's position, especially as a role model for young girls, is quite admirable. Her message is a positive, and necessary, one in a culture that is obsessed with the pursuit of thin at any cost.

Let's be honest, however, Lawrence isn't even close to obese; nor is she overweight. How would culture respond to an obese actress making similar claims? Would she be the on-screen love interest of America's hunks? Would she win the admiration of the masses?

In 2008, while working on the film "Brideshead Revisited," Emma Thompson was protective of a young actress being pressured to lose weight. When Thompson, Oscar-winning actress and screen writer, overheard a producer ask an actress to lose weight, Thompson threatened to quit her job. A subsequent write-up of Thompson's response to her producer's demand of weight loss from other actresses on the set detailed the following rejoinder, "If you speak to her about this again, on any level, I will leave this picture. You are never to do that." Thompson has a long history of opposing the industry's extreme weight pressures, but like many individuals continues to be frustrated at the apparent lack of progress within the industry.

Roseann Barr and Melissa McCarthy have had a very successful career in Hollywood—in part leveraging their physical size to enhance their various roles. They were funny as comedians, and they were also funny as comedians of size. Both women, however, have publicly stated that their weight was one of the greatest struggles that they had experienced and that they did not want to be fat. They fear that not being able to lose their weight could pose medical risk. On the other hand, losing weight could alter public perception of these formerly large and incredibly entertaining actresses.

REDEFINING THE PROBLEM

Our culture views "obesity" as the problem. However, if obesity were the entire problem, then the solution would be to reduce caloric intake and increase caloric expenditure via drugs or exercise. In other words, look at your BMI, set aside the Big Gulp, and then get motivated to lose weight.

Obesity, however, is a reflection of culture, and our culture is part of the problem. The bullying by school children, parents, brand marketers, educators, and even healthcare providers – are part of the culture of obesity, and thus part of what's not working. The obese condition is part of a larger relevant whole and one outward manifestation of a society that often has misinformed expectations and values. Obesity is a manifestation of the problem and not "the problem."

There is no short way home. Addressing obesity begins with redefinition. No one person, alone, can fix the problem, but, collectively, as a culture, with a new collaborative strategy, progress is possible. Healthcare providers can be better informed and can be at the forefront of providing a new direction in addressing this issue. Physicians can end the diet versus no diet debate. Educators and parents, working cooperatively, can facilitate progress. Social and political leaders can address the issues of obesity in all future policies and plans to reduce health risks, not only now, but also in the future. Only then, can we chip away at a culture that celebrates thin, laughs at fat, and disenfranchises generations of obese children and adults.

The way forward is to treat the whole person, rather than the obese condition in isolation. The obese condition does not exist separate from the rest of the individual and that person's community. Furthermore, the condition is not separate from our culture. To reframe the problem of obesity, culture will need to redefine weight-related success and to help individuals, healthcare providers, and our culture be *"UnWeighted"* in living with the issues of obesity. Knowledge must be gained. Trust must be earned. The road is much longer, and the adrenaline of the quick fix is not part of the ride.

"A million little fixes" will be needed to build a nation that is not fixated on weight. This approach will not be contingent on resolving the diet or no diet debate in order to improve physical health and emotional well-being. Success will not be about being skinny or the number of pounds lost. The models on the cover of *Seventeen* will not be photo-shop thin. Success is being able to attend to your health each day and be a healthier person over the course of your lifetime.

UnWeighted Nation sets forth a model for redefining weight-related success. This model will not prescribe the "fix." The new model proposes a self-care process that can occur over a lifetime. It will not have a beginning or an end. There will be no before and after photo. Self-care is a journey that continues over a person's lifetime, leaving a sense of success and accomplishment in each day.

This book advocates a lifelong approach to improving health. Healthcare providers, counselors, educators, and parents all desire the greatest good for our children and our nation's future. In that regard, consider the fact that obesity is the single biggest healthcare challenge in our country since polio. The grave nature of the situation, the issue demands new awareness and new management strategies. The exhausting and futile "diet" or "no diet" debate must end, and new collaborative strategies for improved health must begin.

In reality, changing the way that culture views and treats obesity might seem too insurmountable a task. There are some cultural changes worth fighting for, however. Think of the civil rights movement. Just a little over 50 years ago, Martin Luther King delivered his revolutionary speech. At that time, a majority of Americans rejected civil rights and racial integration. Another segment of the population felt it was an unattainable ideal. There were also some individuals who fought vigilantly, year after year, decade after decade, for racial equality. While racial divides still exist a half decade later, America has made gradual changes to help ensure civil liberties for all races.

Perhaps it's time to join the ranks of healthcare professionals like Natalie Stavas, MD. Yards away from completing her fourth Boston Marathon, she dashed down Hereford Street to aid bomb victims. After this event, she asked, "Why is it that our children are at such a high risk for poor mental health and poor physical health, and are exposed to so much violence? I feel that it is my job as a pediatric physician to find the answer.

How can the obesity crisis be effectively addressed? What cultural changes will enable this goal to be achieved? Those issues are what this book is designed to answer.

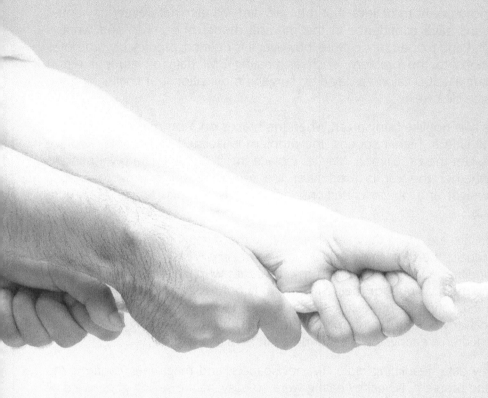

2

It's Not One Thing

"There's no one thing that's true," wrote Ernest Hemingway in *For Whom the Bell Tolls*. "It's all true."

As obesity in America spreads, culture craves the simple, single-truth answer to the epidemic's cause. "Just tell me exactly what I need to do." Or, "Isn't there a pill for this?" Americans want to believe that the next diet will eliminate every unwanted pound. Americans have confidence in the medical model of resolve: find what is broken and fix it. Blind to the truth, culture, however it is defined, predictably promotes simplistic solutions to the problem, such as posting BMI data on student report cards; prescribing a 1500-calorie-a day-diet; surgery; medications; or challenging the hopeful to a juice cleanse.

Fixing obesity is not like fixing a car. When the brakes on a car make noise, or the car pulls to one side at higher speeds, the problem is isolated and fixable. Replace the brake pads. Get the car aligned. Maybe, replace the front tires. The owner knows immediately whether the car is fixed after the repair. Understanding the cause of escalating weight and obese conditions, however, is a much longer and more complex process.

Many Americans are aware they are obese. While the situation may appear obvious for many individuals, the data show that a number of Americans *remain unaware* of their obese condition and the associated risks. Parents who do not have access to regular pediatric medical care for their children, may not realize their infant or child's weight gain is escalating or unhealthy. Furthermore, they may have limited access to good medical advice and/or information to assist them in learning how to best support their children's eating, exercise, and health habits in general.

The monthly data headlining radio, TV, newspapers, and magazines confirms the complexity of the problem. If healthy eating were so easy, as the saying goes, we'd all be doing it. But we're not. In a recent poll, 52 percent of Americans believed doing their taxes was easier than figuring out how to eat healthy.

Like the rhythmic thumping of the bass drum of a marching band, study after study confirms that obesity is worsening. Whatever is being done isn't working, or, at the very least, isn't working well enough to elicit broad and sustained cultural change.

So, what needs fixing? Is it the person's body size? Is it the availability of food? Is it the taste of food? Is it the type of calories consumed? Is it the stress placed on the body because of the increased hours at work? Is it the lack of exercise? Is it the family's gene pool? Is it the lack of discipline or willpower? Or, is it something else?

Most experts agree that it's not one thing. The causes of obesity are multifactorial. The interfacing contributing factors are complex. Without an awareness of what makes obesity so complex, it's tempting to toss around simplistic solutions. On the other hand, it's too late for shallow approaches to stem this global epidemic.

FAST CULTURE

The promise of a quick fix sells in America. Americans crave simplicity and speed. In our fast-paced culture, time is a precious commodity. To "save time," individuals pay more for non-stop air travel, high-speed processors for our computers and mobile devices, and speed passes at amusement parks. To avoid waiting in line, Americans purchase tickets online and pay a premium for overnight delivery. Amazon, the online retailer, is planning to feed American's need for speed when it unrolls its new patent for "anticipatory shipping." This service enables products to be shipped before a buyer actually purchases them. Americans don't have a dime of time to spare. In addition, several restaurants are calculating the predicted number and type of meals, prior to the time of order and making those meals available in neighborhoods and deliverable, within ten minutes of the order being placed.

Individuals in advertising keenly understand this desire for fast: fast is cash. If brand marketers can design a product that promises speed, they will sell more. Take, for instance, the milk carton. More plastic jugs with screw-top lids are sold than cardboard cartons with the press-open spout. Even at a higher price, the plastic jugs are preferred—the perception is faster and easier is better.

A microwaveable lasagna meal promises a "gourmet" meal in half the time. Fast food vendors sell bite-sized fried fish or chicken to reduce the amount of time otherwise needed for cutting, forking, chewing, and multitasking. Why struggle to unwrap two Butterfinger candy bars when you can open one bag of bite-sized Butterfingers and down as many as you would like? Some aluminum cans of beer are currently sold with a second opening on the top surface of the can in order to permit faster and more plentiful pouring and drinking.

With faster-paced dining, food and drink that travel with you, and less-mindful eating circumstances, eating is less well-controlled. Fast sells, and brands grow. In turn, so do our waistlines.

LIFETIME VALUE OF FAST FOOD

Who doesn't like the "fast food" dollar menu or the 2-for-1 food coupon? The underlying marketing strategy is brilliant: lose money on the dollar menu to lure consumers in for the larger margin items. It's about the "lifetime value" of a customer. The availability of cheap, readily available, and densely caloric fast food, however, contributes to obesity in America.

"Fast food is now so commonplace that it is an inevitability," writes Eric Schlosser in *Fast Food Nation: The dark side of the all-American meal*, "as though it were somehow unavoidable, a fact of modern life." He cites that in 1970, Americans spent about $6 billion on fast food. While in 2016, they spent more than $384 billion.

Granted, there are more Americans in 2016 than there were 40 years earlier, but, still, the leap is staggering.

Schlosser points out that more money is spent on fast food than on higher education, personal computers, or new cars. In fact, Americans spend more on fast food than on almost everything. It's simply easy to drop by Wendy's or McDonald's after soccer practice or after mom and dad's long day at work. Fast food has woven its way into the lives of most families. *Fast Food Nation* reported that 12 percent of all Americans have, at one time or another, worked at a McDonalds and that American children now get about one-quarter of their total vegetable servings in the form of potato chips and french fries.

In addition, Schlosser offers a couple of particularly trenchant insights. The first is how fast food targets children. "Fast food is heavily marketed to children," he says, "and prepared by people who are barely older than children. This is an industry that both feeds and feeds off the young." His second insight is what makes it so difficult for parents to wean their kids off fast food: "[Fast food] has been carefully designed to taste good." As such, the consistently flavored chicken nuggets, with the plastic toy, provided in five minutes or less, are the food fare choice of many individuals. Crafty marketing campaigns pair fast-food items with words like "*happy* meal," "*super*-size," "*fun*-pack" and "extra-*value*" to persuade the consumer that they are purchasing something "good."

The frenetic pace of our culture is part of what drives us through the fast food drive-thru rather than to the dinner table. It's why 80 percent of our meals eaten out are not served by a waiter or waitress. Time flies, and so must we, in order to keep pace. Our culture is so fast that it leaves little room for self-sufficiency, let alone the level of self-made, self- care that can result in the drastic weight loss that is so revered by society.

Unless they are contestants on an extreme weight loss show, Americans don't have the time to devote six to ten hours a day to exercise or have the resources to engage trainers, physical therapists, dieticians, and chefs, and provide childcare for the children at home. Yet, this is the type of weight loss that the culture promotes and rewards: fast and drastic. The underlying message for the common person, who slogs away at weight management, day after day, month after month, year after year, is that unless you achieve the "right" size in the "right" time, you are a failure.

As a result, many individuals give up, not realizing that smaller changes, such as increasing their level of fruit and vegetable consumption, or going for a walk, can facilitate weight stability and improve their overall health. Expecting more than one person can achieve and falling short discourages subsequent efforts.

While convenient, tasty, and fun, many processed foods are far from nutritionally ideal. They are densely caloric, as well as higher in sugar, fat, and salt content. Furthermore, they may contain additives and preservatives, and are lacking micro-nutrients that are found in whole grain products, lean proteins, and many fruits and vegetables. In a New York Times article, Hannah Fairfield writes, "No country has embraced the movement toward commercialized, pre-packaged food as much as the United States." She reports that Americans consume 31 percent more packaged foods than fresh food, and that they eat more packaged food per person than those in most other countries." In fact, the largest percent of an American family's grocery bill (23 percent) is spent on processed food and sweets.

The corollary is the added sugar and added fat to the American diet. Americans prefer sugar and sweet-tasting foods and beverages. A report showed that "per capita consumption of caloric sweeteners (dry-weight basis)—mainly sucrose (table sugar made from cane and beets) and corn sweeteners (notably high-fructose corn syrup, or HFCS)—increased 43 pounds, or 39 percent, between 1950-59 and 2000." At the same time that Americans increased their consumption of packaged foods, the portion sizes also increased.

Accordingly, not only is the food less healthy, Americans are eating larger portions of it. With larger portions comes higher daily calorie intake. Between 1971 and 2000, women increased their caloric intake by 22 percent, and men increased theirs by 7 percent. A study by the CDC found a 16 percent increase in sugar consumption by children and adolescents from 2005 to 2008, primarily due to the ingestion of processed foods.

Another study by the CDC discovered a promising 12-year trend among children and adolescents: the number of daily calories ingested by this group had actually decreased. The bad news was these individuals consumed between 11 and 12 percent of their kilocalories from saturated fat. The recommended calories (or kilocalories) from saturated fat is 10 percent. The logical conclusion is that much of the food that is engineered for the palates of our children may not be healthy for them.

While additives, sugar, fat, and larger portions are problematic, environmental factors, such as *food deserts*, complicate the problem further. A food desert is a neighborhood in which there is minimal or limited access to healthy and affordable food, like fresh fruit, vegetables, whole grains, low-fat milk, and other foodstuffs that constitute a healthy diet. The primary source of nutrition in food deserts is often fast food establishments and convenience stores. A government report stated, "Individuals in these areas [food deserts] may be more reliant on convenience, fast food, or similar retailers, or they may not have enough money to afford the higher prices." In contrast, more wealthy communities may have three times as many supermarkets as poor ones do. Furthermore, on average, predominantly Caucasian neighborhoods contain four times as many supermarkets as do predominantly black ones, while grocery stores in African-American communities are generally smaller, with fewer available fruit, vegetable, and healthy food options.

In food desert areas, fast-food chains and convenience stores pick up the slack, offering less expensive "meat," as well as foods that are high in fat, sugar, and salt (e.g., snack cakes, chips, and soda). With more than two percent of all U.S. households living more than a mile away from a supermarket and not owning a car, it's a challenge for many individuals to access healthy, fresh, and seasonal ingredients.

The lack of access to sufficient amounts of food because of limited funds is called *food insecurity*. In fact, more than 49 million American households are considered food insecure and, as a result, they are vulnerable to poor health. With regard to food deserts and food insecurity, the following points help to clarify the relevance of both factors:

- Poverty and food insecurity are related and influence subsequent rates of obesity.
- In 2016, 14 percent of all US households experienced food insecurity, with low-income households, particularly those with children, experiencing household food insecurity at a much higher rate.
- In 2016, 41 percent of low-income households, with children aged six years and younger, in the United States reported low or very- low food security.
- Food insecurity is more common in racial and ethnic minority households (25.1, black; 26.2, Hispanic; and 10.7, Caucasian).
- Women in "very-low or low-security" households are at greater risk of being overweight or obese than women in secure households.
- The effects of low food security or very low food security appear to be meditated by maternal body weight. Persistent household low or very-low security was associated with 22% greater risk of childhood obesity, compared with those individuals who are persistently food secure.
- Among daughters having overweight mothers, greater "eating in the absence of hunger" at age five and greater increases in BMI between ages five and nine years were measured.
- Obese conditions in childhood continue into adulthood.

Too many Americans have minimal access to healthy food. In turn, inadequate access to healthy foodstuffs can diminish the likelihood that a person can consume a healthy diet.

Even if fresh produce were available in food deserts, the issue of obesity would not be resolved. In a provocative article, "How Junk Food Can End Obesity," David H. Freedman discussed whether the availability of healthier food, particularly in food deserts, would help solve the problem of obesity. In short, the answer was no.

The article narrates his journey from his affluent community in the L.A. area to East L.A., with a largely Hispanic population that is "visibly struggling with obesity." He noted the presence of bodegas (convenience stores), which featured fatty meat and canned and boxed foods, shelves of candy and processed snacks, and large displays of sugared beverages. Later, he visited a more vegetable-and-fruit-friendly bodega, which more prominently promoted fruits and vegetables. The store was empty. He writes, "I hung around, eventually buying a few items … finally, a young woman came in and made a beeline for the junk food shelves, grabbed a pack of cupcakes, paid, and left."

Unfortunately, the mere availability of farm-fresh fruits and vegetables alone will not ensure healthy eating. Individuals generally don't change their habits easily. "People aren't going to change their ingrained, neuro-biologically supercharged junk-eating habits," Freedman writes, "just because someone dangles vegetables in front of them, farm-fresh or otherwise." Freedman argues that the whole-foods movement is an emperor with no clothes and that the food industry must design foods with less fat and fewer problem carbohydrates, "trimming unwanted ingredients while preserving the sensations they deliver."

Changing habits or behavior of any kind is typically challenging. Science has shown that ingestion of high-sugar, high-fat, and calorically dense foods increases an individual's desire for these foods. Accordingly, it could be argued that Oreo cookies are more addictive than cocaine. Such a conclusion was confirmed by a 2013 Connecticut College study, which found that Oreo cookies activate more neurons in the pleasure center of a rat's brain than does cocaine. When faced with the choice of hanging out by rice cakes or Oreos, there was no contest. The rats raced to the Oreos. In another test, the rats were given the option of loitering in either an area of the maze in which they would receive a saline injection or another area in which they would receive a shot of cocaine or morphine. Comparatively, the rats craved the Oreo fix as much as the drug.

After exposure to an Oreo, the body craves it—not an apple. After exposure to a Big Mac, the body craves it—not a garden salad. In turn, it becomes harder to satisfy hunger and establish satiety with healthier, but less densely caloric, food items. As a result, individuals pass through the drive-thru for more of the same.

SCREEN TIME

If ubiquitous, low-cost, engineered-to-taste-great and make-you-feel-happy fast food were not enough, data from the World Health Organization indicates that other factors are in play that also contribute to the obesity crisis. For example, 60 to 85 percent of people in the world—from both developed and developing countries—lead sedentary lifestyles. The phrase sedentary lifestyle refers to those individuals who do little physical activity or no relatively vigorous exercise (such as running, calisthenics, swimming, tennis, etc. In fact, most of the individuals in this segment of the population barely partake in activities that could be classified as moderate-intensity (e.g., walking, gardening, golf, etc.). In the U.S., watching TV ranks only behind work and sleep as the most commonly reported activities. In fact, watching television encompasses just over half of all of the average person's leisure time.

Some economists have attempted to calculate the cost of inactivity, connecting a sedentary lifestyle to direct medical spending. The resultant number, which is in the 10s of billions, rises each year. Even more disturbing is the astounding fact that it is estimated that physical inactivity is responsible for almost 200,000 or 1 in 10 deaths each year.

Evidence shows that the amount of time that the average kid spends watching a screen during the course of the day correlates with a rise in obesity, as well as an increase in metabolic risk factors in children. In turn, this situation has contributed to an increase in heart disease, type 2 diabetes, asthma, and, among other factors, sleep apnea in kids. Stanford University pediatrician, Thomas N. Robinson, estimates that up to 25 percent of the food-intake time of children happens while watching television. The more TV that children watch, the more likely they are to gain excess weight. Furthermore, kids who have TV sets in their bedrooms gain even more excess weight than those children who don't. It appears that TV habits in childhood ripple throughout their life and are a predictor of obesity in adulthood.

Madison Avenue, as well as the brands it represents, has benefited substantially from children's increased screen time. A young, malleable, and captive audience watches hundreds of food-related ads each year. The screen, the jingles, the colorful packaging, and the snacks tend to mesmerize kids. Marketers use the phrase "pester power" to describe how their messages influence kids to cajole their parents to buy branded products.

In reality, many of the branded foods, drinks, and restaurants promoted during programming for children are unhealthy. A study of food brands appearing in prime-time television programming in 2008 found that children and teens saw roughly one food brand per day, and three out of four of these brand appearances were for sugary soft drinks. Given the ever-expanding number of product placements, including in digital goods, it is obvious that advertising works. For example, one experiment showed that children who watched cartoons with food commercials ate 45 percent more snack food while viewing, than children who watched cartoons with non-food advertising.

It may be that the exposure children to food ads does more damage than the inactivity of TV watching itself. One study tracked the TV habits and change in BMI of 1,100 young children over a five-year period. The study compared those children who watched TV with commercials and those kids who viewed TV with no commercials. As it turned out, the more hours per day of commercial TV children watched at the start of the study, the more likely they were to have a relative increase in BMI at the study's end. On the other hand, among kids who watched non-commercial TV, there was no correlation with change in their BMI.

While screen time slows metabolism, and commercials encourage consumption of densely caloric food consumption, television producers pair laugh tracks with weight-related discriminatory images. A study conducted at the University of Minnesota found that 37 percent of television programming for children and teens depicted images of overweight individuals in a disparaging manner. The heavier individual was the subject of a joke or teasing. The smaller individuals were depicted in more successful, attractive or powerful roles. Not only does such an environment encourage weight gain, it also simultaneously denigrates children and teens of size.

Overall, findings suggest that youth are exposed to instances of weight stigmatization from an early age and in a format that conveys that these behaviors are socially acceptable. Furthermore, such programming sends a message that an individual's body is not good enough, regardless of shape or size—an idea that contributes to body dissatisfaction amongst youngsters. To provide informed programming that will accurately shape the public's understanding and attitudes about body weight, shape, and size, the following actions, as identified by the "Guidelines for Media Portrayals for Individuals Affected by Obesity" (collaboratively developed by the Rudd Center for Food Policy and Obesity, Obesity Action Coalition and The Obesity Society) are recommended:

- Individuals affected by excess weight should be depicted in various roles including ones of authority, expertise, intelligence, and competence. Negative stereotypes depicting people in larger bodies as lazy, weak, stupid, or targets of humor should be avoided.
- Weight-related humor that may perpetuate negative assumptions regarding size, weight, and/or shape should be avoided.
- Weight-stigmatizing comments should not be met with audience laughter or neutrality.
- The use of images that depict overweight or obese individuals as either disheveled or wearing revealing clothing should be avoided. Undue influence on specific body parts should also be avoided.
- Undue emphasis on weight should be avoided.

DRIVERS OF INACTIVITY

Stress is a staple of modern life. Statistics indicate that many Americans medicate their stress with a higher fat diet, less exercise, and more smoking. Furthermore, animal studies show that when animals in a zoo are bored or stressed, they either eat too much or stop eating. A similar eating pattern for humans (i.e., eating too much) results in higher storage of abdominal fat, a marker for increased health risk. Stress can also lead to emotional eating, which, in turn, only leads to more stress and weight gain.

In America, kids feel stressed. They feel pressured to be leaders, to be captains of their teams, and to excel at everything they try. They feel that they must be and do more. As a result, they undertake what they consider to be proactive steps, such as, taking advanced placement classes, studying late into the night for top grades, joining the debate team, serving as captain of a varsity sport, volunteering for community service, and anything else that "looks good on paper"—just to enhance the likelihood that they will meet college admissions requirements and be ensured a "successful" future.

Recently a room full of high school juniors, immersed in the college application process was asked how much stress they were feeling on a scale of zero to 100. Many replied "120-150."

Locked into so many obligations, they have little time or freedom to explore their lives and discover who they are. Their identity may be defined predominantly by the expectations and roles assigned to them by the culture and other people. They are less and less able to discover and freely elect for themselves who they are.

Parents can lose sight of the possibilities of a growth process that can be more empowering, healthy, and fulfilling for their children. More often than not, parents get caught in the "more is better" trap. More homework falsely promises smarter. More expensive college, falsely promises better education. More after-school activities, falsely promises a more "well-rounded," emerging adult. As a result, children lose much in this process. Unfortunately, many children do not have the down time necessary for recovery from stress and the development of a clear sense of identity needed to become healthy adults.

One way that humans recover from stress is through play. Play is that activity which occurs without goal or product. It is largely unstructured time. Physical activity may be playful, if it is unfettered by structure. It's what happens at the park, at the pool, or in the neighbor's backyard. Kicking a ball is playful. As a rule, soccer team practice, for example, more often than not, is not play, especially when there is pressure to win, the practice is structured, and the demands of the endeavor are endless. Pass, trap, cross, shoot, ad infinitum!

Both play and physical activity are necessary to cope with stress and to be healthy children and adults. Studies show that animals that have had sufficient and enjoyable physical activity are more resilient when faced with mental stressors (e.g., loud sounds or crowded conditions) than those that have little physical activity. Furthermore, animals that are more physically fit, in the face of stress, have less production of cortisol (a stress hormone) than those that are unfit.

Cortisol is a hormone produced by the adrenal glands as part of an individual's daily hormonal cycle, typically in response to the body's fight-or-flight mechanism. If the demands of life become too intense (resulting in stress), the body secretes cortisol, which, in turn results in an increase in appetite. Not surprisingly, over time, the body's system of hormonal checks and balances can, to a degree, promote weight gain, given the fact that rarely does a stressed-out lifestyle lead to healthy eating habits.

Despite the benefits of being physically fit as a result of engaging in physical activity on a regular basis, as touted by national media-driven campaigns like Play 60 and Let's Move, America's children are playing less and watching TV more. A survey conducted by the YMCA found that 74 percent of parents say they choose to spend family time with their children sitting in front of a TV set. The same survey also revealed that "74 percent of children between the ages of 5 and 10 do not get enough exercise on a daily basis, based on the 60 minutes of daily physical activity recommended in the government's Physical Activity Guidelines for Americans." In addition, 42 percent of parents indicated that technological distractions (i.e., screen time) get in the way of active play. In reality, less than 50 percent of high schools students reported that they attended physical education classes in an average week while in school. While numerous potential solutions exist, no one person or group is armed to cut the Gordian knot alone.

EATING OUT: THE PERFECT STORM

Whether dining in restaurants or eating at school, the more an individual eats out, the more likely they are to be overweight. Like other environmental factors, this situation contributes to the perfect storm, one in which Americans are eating out more and more. In fact, a study by the U.S. Department of Agriculture reported that a third of all calories consumed by Americans now come from outside the home.

One problematic component of eating out is the content of the food—more sugar and more fat. Another factor is the portion size. A bagel from 20 years ago was much smaller and contained 140 calories. Many bagels from some of the top current brands, like Panera, contain 290 calories or more, which is two times the energy content previously seen.

"For the average consumer," says Lisa Mancino, a food economist for the USDA, "eating one meal away from home each week translates to roughly two extra pounds a year." In reality, a number of Americans eat out more often than once a week. For Americans with kids in school, restaurant eating after basketball or football practice, for example, is a ritual that often happens more than once a week. Eating out has become a form of survival; dinner is one less thing to manage in a stress-filled day.

While chain restaurants were recently required in 2015 to post calories on their menus, calorie counts on their bill of fare do little to change behavior. In fact, for some individuals, having the caloric counts of the various items on the menus, as well as having access to additional nutritional information, might not change their meal choices in a healthy direction. They still choose food with higher calories. For other individuals, seeing the caloric information may cause them to experience an increased level of anxiety. Studies indicate that calorie count for an item may become a reason to choose something else. "People expect something to taste worse, if they believe it is healthy," writes David H. Freedman.

The school lunch is a form of eating out. At the present time, American schools provide breakfast and lunch to 31 million children. The program is an easy target. The topic of school lunches has spawned a couple awarding-winning short films, including *Yuck: A 4th Grader's Short Documentary about School Lunches* and *Lunch*. In *Yuck*, Zachary Maxwell surreptitiously documents his public school lunch experience and concludes that much of it is processed food. Voila! His documentary wins a couple of awards.

While some progress has been made to reduce caloric content and increase the amount of fresh fruits and vegetables in school lunches, the average school lunch still contains more than 800 calories, or more than half of what some children need throughout an entire day. For example, an inactive middle-school girl may need only 1400 to 1600 calories per day.

The a la carte menu at many schools poses another problem. Susan Levin, director of nutrition education for the Physicians Committee for Responsible Medicine, believes that the food pyramid, which was created by the USDA and is no longer used by that agency, favored the interests of the agricultural industry. According to Levin, there's too much fat in the menu. Furthermore, Levin goes on, "The USDA is paying industry— huge corporations—for their overproduced goods." In addition, at least 20 percent of schools also sell fast food, such as Taco Bell, Pizza Hut, and Little Caesars. Collectively, these conditions constitute a huge challenge for our children.

THE INHERITED HUMAN BODY

"I don't think obesity is a disease," he said. He is a 54-year-old executive who does hot yoga four times a week and looks as fit as he was in high school. It's hard for him, as it is for many Americans to imagine why someone is obese. Like many Americans, he is unaware of another significant contributor to obesity—an individual's gene pool.

For many individuals, genetics and biology are more influential than all the other factors previously discussed—combined. It's easy to believe that overeating and inactivity alone cause obesity. It should be noted, however, that people who are thin also overeat on occasion. In addition, some individuals who are inactive can be thin as well.

In a cab recently, in Las Vegas, the driver was asked about his favorite local restaurants and food items. He excitedly declared that his favorite meal was mashed potatoes, served under a thick layer of duck fat. As a driver, it was assured that he spent many hours daily sitting, a relatively sedentary occupation. When he jumped out at the end of the drive to help with the door, he appeared to be approximately six feet tall, 40 to 50 years of age, and very, very thin. It was a reminder that obese conditions may not develop if other factors, such as genetics and biology, successfully counter such a transformation.

Even thin people are at the mercy of their gene pool. Given the right genetic variant, individuals can be thin, but still prone to high levels of cholesterol and diabetes. In other words, a person may have the genetic propensity to be "thin," but sufficient and repeated exposure to high caloric intake and low caloric expenditure can alter genetics, and contribute to the development of obese conditions.

Consider the study by Li and his coworkers who developed a genetic predisposition score, based on the weighted effect of 12 genetic markers. Researchers studied the association between this genetic predisposition score and the BMI of 20,430 Caucasian men and women. For each increment in the score, an increase occurred in BMI that was equivalent to 1.0 pound for a person 67 inches tall. In other words, there is a genetic predisposition to being overweight.

It is interesting to note that while an inactive person at the same height had an increase of 1.3 pounds for each increment in the scale, an active person had an increase of only 0.8 pounds. Therefore, even though a genetic predisposition to obesity exists, a physically active lifestyle was associated with a 40 percent reduction in that risk.

The weight status of parents has an impact on their kid's weight. For example, statistics show that there is a 79 percent risk of obesity in 10- to 14-year-olds, if one parent is obese. It's difficult to know whether this factor is a byproduct of the living environment, the inherited genes, or both factors combined.

Studies show that about 30 to 40 percent of the variance in caloric and macronutrient intake among spouses, parents, and children is associated with genetic influences.

Recent neuroimaging research confirms that neurochemistry has a powerful impact on such factors as eating behavior, hunger, satiety, thoughts of food, thoughts of eating, and urges to eat. The relationship between neurochemistry and obesity appears to be reciprocally related, but understanding the specific processes is still in the embryonic stage. The pathways are complex, and much more needs to be understood.

Studies based on animal models are informing the discipline. For example, levels of the hormone leptin appear to influence reactivity to images of food and self- reported "liking of food." Several scientists likened the neurochemical patterns to those seen in addictions to cocaine. Neurochemical changes, in the form of altered dopamine D2 receptors (D2R), create reward hyposensitivity and drive the development of compulsive eating. Eating patterns, themselves, may further alter neurochemistry in ways that aggravate eating behavior and contribute to the obese condition. In other words, compulsive eating behavior itself may have neurochemical properties that are powerfully influential and require careful evaluation and intervention.

SLOWING DOWN

In order to be more successful when addressing the issue of obesity, a more deliberate approach may be required, at least initially. Such an approach necessitates greater consideration of the complexity of obesity, changed attitudes and abandoned assumptions about individuals of all sizes. Instead of darting out to buy the latest diet book or signing up, in January, yet again, for one of the branded diet plans, maybe it's time to slow down, approach this issue with caution, and consider the vast array of alternatives.

What healthy eating approach may best fit your teenager, whose eating is predominantly elsewhere—with neighbors, or friends, at school, or restaurants, etc.? How does lecturing your children work? Should you lock up your food, in the hope that your children will be more disciplined (i.e., consume healthy food) in what they eat? The issue, however, is more complex than parents giving reminders about eating right, and kids just saying "no." What do you say, when your 13-year-old son finally blurts out what he has been thinking for some time, "Don't you think I know anything? Do you think I'm stupid? Do you think that I don't care? That I don't try?" By now, he has heard the message that "fat is bad" and perhaps he has come to the conclusion that "he is bad too."

It's not that parents shouldn't do something. Parents are and will continue to do lots of things. For all too often, however, parents continue to feel defeated and hopeless about helping their kids learn to take care of themselves? The situation is further compounded by a multi-billion dollar weight loss industry, which includes products, books, TV shows, marketing, and advertising. Arguably, everyone benefits from a greater level of awareness concerning the physical and emotional risks of traditional dieting. On the other hand, what we are doing might not be helpful. In fact, it may be making it worse. We want "the" fix and there isn't "one."

One viable place to start is developing a keen awareness of environmental factors that perpetuate obesity uniquely for each individual. Perhaps, both parents work, or a single mom is raising three kids, mostly on her own and without abundant free time to plan, shop for, and prepare family meals. It might be difficult to walk to school, given the morning schedules of kids, from kindergarten to a senior in high school. Maybe, the route to school is dangerous, the weather is inclimate, or the sidewalks are unavailable or in poor repair. Financial circumstances may limit food quality and availability. As a result, the half-mile of physical activity and healthy home-cooked family meal that may benefit children, are not always feasible or even possible. The point is that obesity is not caused by a single factor. Each person's current picture and path moving forward is unique. Health- and weight-related matters tend to be complex and ever-evolving. Therefore, the shortest path to curbing obesity is not a one-step solution.

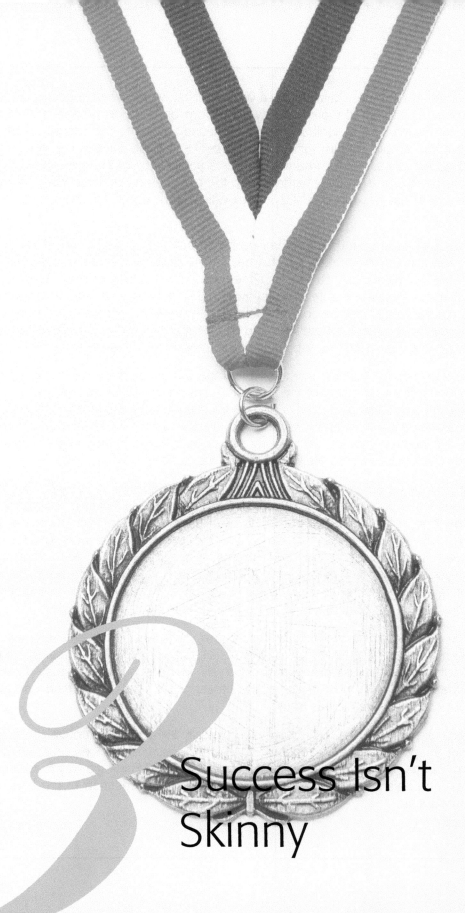

Success Isn't Skinny

He wore his green t-shirt like Miss America wears her crown. A senior executive of a major corporation, "Rick" had worked his way up from obscurity to prominence. He was known for his intellect, as well as his strategic contributions to the success of the company that had employed him for over a decade. He was devoted to his wife and contributed generously to his community. He was a paragon of success, except when it came to his health. Outside the boardroom, to the common cultural observer, it was wrongly assumed that he appeared lazy, weak-willed, and a flop. He was morbidly obese at 595 pounds.

Hundreds of excess pounds compromised his health and choked his confidence. Walking 15 feet left him breathless and his back in pain. Swollen feet made slipping on his shoes a herculean task. Lacing his shoes was off the list of options. Breaking chairs in public places was a real fear. When traveling, he requested a hotel room with a handicap bathroom because he couldn't hoist his legs over the edge of a tub or turn around in a regular shower. Impossible to find clothes that fit him, he had them tailor-made. A less encumbered life was slipping away with each pound gained.

"You have to change," his boss insisted. His company mandated that he lose weight, after he no longer fit into the seat of the company's private jet. While change is easy to mandate, it is difficult to effect. At nearly 600 pounds, the idea of losing even 10 pounds felt like anticipating a Mount Kilimanjaro climb. Losing 100 pounds would not equate to "not obese." He would not appear slim. Losing 100 pounds would not mean guaranteed applause from his doctor or boss. He would still be obese, so why try?

Fearing job loss, he enlisted support. He arranged for meals to be delivered to avoid the ubiquitous larger-portioned restaurant dining. His wife agreed to be supportive by changing the kinds of foods they kept at home. He signed on for therapy to help identify and understand the "why" of his weight. He learned how painful emotions related to early trauma were quickly and completely wiped away by food. Thinking about food, cooking, planning meals, eating, and feeling full all helped to push away his tormenting past. Sweet foods, salty, crunchy, dense, and abundant food provided emotional sustenance … temporarily. He struggled to learn new ways to cope.

He hired a personal trainer, despite having low confidence in their usefulness. Trainers often did not want to work with people of size or feel adept in safely and effectively guiding their exercise regimen. After all, he was quickly exhausted in navigating the painful walk to the door of the fitness facility, with little or no energy remaining for exercise once he was inside.

Exercise was painful. All of it. This situation typically led to a trip through the fast food drive-in for post-work-out compensatory eating. Most common exercises were beyond him. Sit-ups? No way. Not one rep. A bench press? No. Finding a way to recline to the bench and balance long enough to complete a single repetition of the bench press was impossible.

Seating surfaces in most exercise facilities did not accommodate size. Given that most exercise specialists are not formally trained to work with a "deconditioned or obese population," they quickly become discouraged. Collectively, these factors only further add to his mounting frustration and shame.

When the trainer arrived at his front door on *"this first day,"* he said "nice to meet you—let's go take a walk," Rick was terrified. "Aren't we going to talk first?"

"We can talk, while we walk. Let's go." By the time they reached the mailbox—not even 15 feet away—Rick's fear manifested as a spasm stabbing his lower back. Defeat swept over him. Here we go again. The trainer showed him an exercise to stretch out his back, and the pain disappeared. "How did you do that?" Rick asked. Instead of fear and discomfort ending the exercise for the day, they paused to stretch and breathe. They then proceeded for another 15 feet … and another … and another. This time, fatigue did not end the exercise session. This time, fatigue did not mean failure. Instead, fatigue meant pausing to recollect and then to continue exercising.

Performing intermittent or discontinuous exercise, which some trainers advocate, provides many of the health benefits achieved by continuous exercise activity. Unfortunately, its benefits are not always appreciated. On occasion, participants can be left feeling unnecessarily insufficient or not good enough, especially when they're comparing their own activities with those of others. The important point to keep in mind, particularly in this situation, is that while less may be different, it is not necessarily less successful.

"I didn't do it. You did it," his trainer responded. Over a four-year period, Rick managed to lose almost 300 pounds. By definition, however, he was still obese. On the other hand, after achieving his first 50-pound loss, he could breathe more comfortably, get up to use the restroom without assistance, get through the day with more energy, and move more freely and with less fear of pain or immobility.

Success or failure? By the time that his weight loss had reached 100 pounds (an amount of weight most people can't even lift), he was able to walk a half mile. Success or failure? At the point when he had lost 300 pounds, he was able to get through the day without sweating through his clothes. He was also able to sleep more comfortably, experience less back and joint pain, and have intimate relations with his wife. In addition, he was able to walk without assistance to the furthest airport terminal. In the process, a sense of confidence and independence that he had not known for years had returned. He was still obese, however. Did his numbers tell the whole story?

His trainer celebrated Rick's triumphs. He bought him a green 6X-large t-shirt, which was many sizes smaller than the one that Rick had previously worn. "What you've accomplished," said his trainer, "is honored by presenting you with this green t-shirt."

Proudly, he wore that green t-shirt until it was rag-frayed, stretched, and potted with holes. Frankly, he wouldn't have cared as much had he been given a Bentley. The t-shirt marked an accomplishment that money couldn't buy. An emerging "internal" strength and sense of accomplishment fueled his continued commitment to himself.

He felt "successful" in any number of many ways. Sadly, however, the public might glance his way, regard his existing shape, make assumptions, and wonder why he "just doesn't try harder."

ENDLESS CYCLE

Everyone needs recognition. Everyone wants to feel successful. Imagine the frustration that individuals might face when hearing, "You lost 75 pounds. Just 75 more to go!" During a recently attended social event, a small group of adults were overheard commenting on the noticeable weight loss of an adult male in his mid-60s. He had just arrived at the party and was shedding his outer coat. Some in attendance were keenly aware of the behind-the-scenes effort that he had made to achieve this much change. He was exercising, monitoring his caloric intake, taking dance lessons, asking his wife to help with preparation of healthy meals, and repeatedly managing the expense psychotherapy support, and new clothes to accommodate his ever-changing size.

His body size was changing dramatically. As a result, he had the pressure of others possibly noticing. The escalating fear of relapse that could lead to further public judgment was palpable. "Wow, one woman commented, Steven looks great." Another male said, "I heard he lost 75 pounds." In this small circle, sipping on drinks prior to the evening's main event another replied, "Yea, imagine how good he would look if he lost 75 more."

Her words were infuriating, but, unfortunately not surprising or problematic for the small circle of individuals who were overheard. Her words represent a culture fixated on appearance and ideals. She is the product of a culture that recreationally scrutinizes celebrity cellulite, thigh gaps, and belly bulges. She has little awareness of actual weight-related challenges and complexities. She does not know that "thinness" is not always a barometer for good health and life satisfaction.

The specific definitions of success and failure serve as the foundation of a traditional diet mentality. Success is commonly understood to mean losing all the excess weight. Success is forever keeping off all the pounds lost. Success is understood as reaching and maintaining an ideal weight. The reward is delivered when the scale settles on the ideal number, or when you fit into your smallest pair of blue jeans, or when friends or anyone else says to you, "See how amazing you look!" The traditional diet mentality targets quantifiable results like, scaled weights, height/weight charts, Kcals, and clothing size. Self-care, effort, and the tenacity to improve health are less regarded and, as such, often not valued or even noticed.

Our culture equates success with power, beauty, and perfection that are narrowly defined. Americans are obsessed with physical perfection. Advertisers know that pairing any product, albeit an automobile, perfume, or beer with a thin body, will boost sales. Good-looking political candidates have the winning edge even before they speak. In one study, participants were asked to predict who would win an instrumental music contest, based on appearance alone, never having heard the musician perform. Looks alone were highly correlated with winning.

Americans fixate on appearance, often remembering the details of someone's outfit or hairstyle over the details of a conversation or personal history, Popular television shows highlight fashion do's and don'ts, offer styling options, and feature before and after images of celebrities and more. Many secretly enjoy the tabloid's headline "Best Beach Bodies" and delight when someone makes the "Worst Beach Body" list. "The Learning Channel" knows that people will tune in when they produce a series called "My 600 Pound Life," a documentary overview of people struggling to lose weight. It's also why "The Biggest Loser" continues to pull in millions of viewers, even after 15 seasons.

When the confetti falls on "The Biggest Loser," the contestants who have been eliminated fade into obscurity. Their blood pressure may be lower. They may be able to finally go on a hike with their family. They may even feel good about their not-yet-perfect physique. On the other hand, they're not the "biggest" loser. They are just the "loser." More often than not, the audience applauds the thinnest, and the runner-ups disappear. Subsequently, a new get-thin-quick spokesperson is born. Thin appears to win again.

American culture champions the "before-and-after" story. A simple Google search, "What is weight-loss success?" yields page after page of "I did it!" feats, with pre- and post-weight loss bikini pics. Not surprisingly, the diet industry (e.g., Atkins, Weight Watchers, Jillian Michael's 30-Day Shred, etc.) sponsors many of these before-and-after forums. Surprisingly, many health-and-fitness magazines, like *Fitness, Health, Shape,* and *Prevention*, do, too.

In a number of ways, these "feel-great-look-great" weight-loss stories are an extension of the $60+ billion dieting industry that champions get-fit-quick diets and workouts for a sculpted, fatless body. In an article entitled "'Weigh Less, Smile More: How Fitness Magazines Define Health in Very Unhealthy Ways," the author, Lindsay Kite, points out that content in these magazines consistently focuses less on overall health and wellness and more on "fast weight loss and the easiest way to get looking sexy." Furthermore, she argues that these magazines dangerously re-package the thin ideal. "Concepts like 'your best body ever' and 'your better-body goals' are combined with straightforward messages advocating daily weight loss; [these magazines] continue to equate thinness with self-improvement and fitness achievement—for every reader, regardless of size or weight."

Accordingly, when you eventually look like Carrie Underwood, after she follows a 20-pound slim-down plan, then you can smile. Then, you're photo-ready. Simply stated, then, you are labeled a success.

For many individuals, however, such success is either fleeting or unattainable. In fact, reaching for "ideal" only frustrates the weight-loss process. Over 10 years ago, Kelly Brownell, internationally renowned expert on obesity, in an article that appeared in *U.S. News and World Report*, "The Science of Slimming," pointed out that "one major way of undermining motivation is to expect more than you can accomplish ... the challenge is to help people be happy with a modest weight loss and maintain it over time."

Weight loss isn't an easy or simple process, when you factor in cultural, genetics, environmental, and physiological influences. "The body is malleable to some degree, but certainly not to the degree suspected by the public," writes Brownell. "It is my belief that many individuals have biological barriers that determine a lower limit for weight, along with limits for how much body shape can change."

In reality, how easily and how much weight a person can actually lose is often predetermined by such factors as physiology, genetics, biology, dieting history, etc. Human bodies are calibrated to hover around a "set point." For some individuals, that set point is lower than for others. Set-point theory suggests that internal regulators, like metabolism or the appetite-suppressing hormones, such as Leptin, adjust when we starve or overeat to protectively regulate weight.

Dieting, can change chemicals and enzymes that influence the intensity of hunger and/or fat storage. This is the body's natural way of protecting itself and preventing additional weight loss. It's no wonder when a dieter is starving, all they can think about is a cheeseburger and Oreo cookies. They are hungry. As such, that's often the types of foods they reach for and ultimately consume. Not surprisingly, many individuals who lose weight will struggle to maintain those weight losses. For a time, dieters may master the scale, but, eventually, the appetite fights back in a powerful manner.

Patterns of weight cycling, with repeated patterns of gains and loss, are associated with an emotional and chemical rollercoaster that can impair the best efforts to maintain a healthy or stable weight. Figure 3-1 exemplifies this pattern. When an individual feels "fat" and the cultural expectation is "thin," they are more likely to diet. Diet is thought to be the cultural cure-all. Hunger signals may return with a vengeance. Exercise regimens may need to be intensified or modified to sustain weight loss.

Relatively few individuals, however, can muster the willpower to win the standoff with hunger. Gradually, the weight may come back. Frustration ensues. In turn, the dieters increase how much they eat in response to trying to manage their levels of screaming hunger and frustration. The cycle repeats. Sadly, the evidence shows that the greater number of diet attempts in a person's history is associated with subsequent greater rapid weight gain, often ending in a higher weight than that which preceded the onset of the diet in the first place.

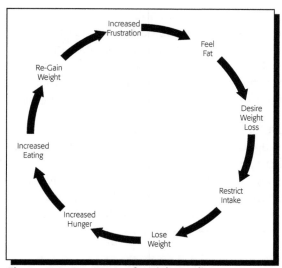

Figure 3-1. A pattern of weight-cycling

What would drive someone to such a life-sucking cycle? In her article that appeared in an issue of *Behavior Therapy*, "Dieting and the Search for the Perfect Body: Where Physiology and Culture Collide," Kelly Brownell addressed this diet mentality, which is built on two false notions perpetuated by culture. First, that when prescribed the right combination of diet and exercise, anyone can reach the thin ideal. Second, once that goal is reached "vast rewards await that person." Not everyone, however, can reach that ideal and sustain that weight. For those individuals who do reach their ideal weight-loss goal, the rewards, he points out, are often less than expected.

While improved health is one possible reward, it may not be as much of a motivator for healthy eating and exercise as the promise of what thinness represents. Improved health, research shows, is not a powerful motivator for healthy eating and more exercise. Most people are also not highly motivated for a number of health-related behaviors, such as taking prescribed blood pressure medicine regularly, flossing teeth daily, completing an entire course of antibiotics, stopping smoking, etc., even when they are aware that the benefits could be improved health.

The factors that prompt an individual to start exercising on a regular basis are usually quite different from those factors which continue an exercise regimen. In oversimplified terms, many people begin their physical activity program because of factors that originate outside themselves (e.g., external reasons). For example, some individuals want to improve how their body, shape, or appearance is viewed by others. Others become physically active because they perceive exercising as the "trendy" thing to be seen doing. A number of people exercise simply because they are told it will improve their health. Still others exercise because someone they know, such as their physician, family, or friends, advised them to do so.

These same people, however, will continue to exercise for reasons that are more "internal". For example, some are motivated to continue because their participation was enjoyable or because they experienced improvement in factors they valued such as posture, energy, or mobility. Still others are motivated by enjoying the social aspects of exercise and physical activity. The point to remember is that individuals start, continue with, or drop out of their exercise programs for their own personal reasons.

One recently conducted study concerning exercise adherence, found that the attendance of middle-aged men was much better if the person's spouse or significant other in his life (i.e., boss, friends, co-workers, etc.) were positive about his participation. In other words, receiving positive support from those individuals who are perceived as important to the exerciser, is key to a person's continued participation. On the other hand, when individuals feel rigid rules and requirements are imposed upon them, their level of motivation for exercise declines.

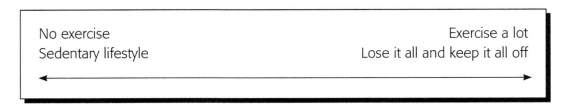

Beauty, power, and success appear to be powerful motivators in the early phases of change. To the outside world, the perfect body signals hard work, self-control, ambition, and power. People who are relatively thin, in comparison to their counterparts, are more likely to earn more, more likely to be hired, more likely to be selected for friendship, and more likely to be seen as successful. To embrace that notion is to also believe in the converse: being overweight suggests laziness and a weak will.

The problem is that many dieters, as do people, fall short of the ideal. Either that or they experience brief joy, while enjoying the admiration of others around them. On occasion, they celebrate their success by eating more. Low-calorie diets, however, tend to feel depriving. Furthermore, frequent and intense exercise can be challenging to sustain. Diets end. Portion sizes increase. The ban on restricted foods is lifted. Subsequently, the treadmill returns to its role as a convenient clothesline.

THE MYTH OF THE NUMBER'S REWARD

Weight-related success can feel elusive. People may believe that reaching "that preselected number" will bring greater "satisfaction" than it does. Some believe, "If I can just get to this weight, or this size, then I will "look" the way I want to look, as well as be happy and in control." On the other hand, when asked, what would "this happy" look like or what would it be like to have all you desire, the answers vary. For example, "I would be liked by others." "I would be respected." "I would be accepted by my family and friends." "I would receive the admiration and respect that I see others receive." "I would be more social." Finally, "I would like myself."

It is important to be aware that numbers on a scale or on a chart do not always ensure outcomes like respect, control, social ability, or happiness. For those individuals who find their way to a lower weight and realize they have not found the respect, control, and happiness they were seeking, two things often happen: 1) a new and even lower weight goal is established, or 2) weight escalation begins. The key point is that weight change alone does not always mean that an individual is able to find the happiness they expect, desire, and deserve.

The medical community frequently thinks about health and weight in terms of body mass index (BMI). To members of this group, such numbers simply define success.

In a different context, a number of experts on higher education also recently turned to *numbers* in an effort to define success. In September 2013, *Time Magazine* organized a summit to discuss the future of higher education. As the cost of higher education continues to increase, so do questions about its value. Will college graduates be able to produce wealth upon graduation? How prepared will they be for the workforce?

As such, ongoing uncertainty exists concerning about which curriculum is ideal. For example, some individuals are for a humanities-oriented curriculum, or a science and math-oriented curriculum. Others advocate for the implementation of a core curriculum, or the implementation of a specialized curriculum. To a degree, the list of possible focal points is somewhat extensive. U.S. Secretary of Education, Arne Duncan, argues for the development of a rating system to help keep colleges and universities "accountable" and to demonstrate the "value" of higher education.

Duncan's interest in a "rating system" is analogous to the fascination with the BMI ratings. Numbers seem to offer some measure of reassurance. Focusing on the numbers provides some individuals with a sense that they have the 411 on what's happening. Generating a number, monitoring any change in a number, and comparing numbers help make most activities, including education and weight control, feel somewhat manageable.

Numbers are visible. They can be compared and tracked. On the other hand, an interpretation of numbers alone has limitations. A rating system for undergraduate education, for example, cannot accurately represent a student's entire scholastic experience or completely predict a student's future success. Similarly, a number on a BMI chart does not capture a person's entire health story. For example, because BMI doesn't account for varying proportions of fat and muscle, it doesn't accurately differentiate between the body compositions of an athletic and non-athletic body types.

Athletic and muscular bodies can elevate BMI. It should also be noted that BMI, alone, does not depict a person's history of dieting or weight change or stability.

Accordingly, a downward change in the BMI percentile does not provide an accurate indication of how that weight change was attained. For example, while healthy exercise can account for some downward adjustment in BMI, a bad recreational drug habit can also lower it. Furthermore, BMI calculations cannot always accurately account for the specifics of each person's overall health. Experts have concluded that some people can have excess fat and be healthy, just as some people can be skinny and unhealthy. It is important to realize that BMI alone does not gauge the physiological, psychological, cultural, and environmental factors that all impact a person's health story.

Straight A's in school do not guarantee future happiness. Being highly paid in your company does not insure respect. Winning the popular vote in one election does not promise future popularity. By the same token, defining success by a BMI chart does not guarantee good health or optimal body size. According to the renowned exercise physiologist, Steven Blair, and relative to the risk of developing cardiovascular disease, it is better to be overweight and exercising, than skinny and not exercising.

Implicitly, culture promises that the more control you have of your weight, the more control you will have of your life. However, the life stories of Americans are full of so many more antagonists than just their weight. Young people navigate the tortuous road to adulthood with broken hearts, peer pressure, addictions, insisting parents, academic stress, and the disappointment when they don't make varsity. Adults still deal with lost jobs, upside-down mortgages, ailing parents, frustrated children, and the perceived betrayal by friends and colleagues, as well as cancer and other debilitating diseases.

However, great risk exists in defining success in numbers. The numbers don't reflect the whole picture. A diet may "fix" your weight (if only briefly), but it doesn't fix your life. In fact, it might actually create more problems. When a University of Minnesota researcher looked at adolescent girls in different treatment groups, she found that five to seven years later, those individuals who focused the most on diet, weight loss, calorie reduction, and exercise gained weight and were at a higher risk for eating disorders. The earlier someone is exposed to a diet-controlled mentality, e.g., diet drinks, weight-loss shakes, calorie-charting, exercise for the purpose of caloric expenditure, and the belief that thin is the ideal that must be pursued at all costs, the greater their likelihood of becoming obese and the greater their degree of obesity in adulthood. The diet's broken promise betrays dieter after dieter.

Obsession with thinness can also lead to a less satisfying life. Many individuals who are dieting are plagued by fear, once they reach their "number." Their minds are hives, buzzing with calculations: What can I eat? When can I eat? When and how much should I exercise? What will happen if I miss Spinning class? If I don't run my six miles, will I gain weight? Will I stop exercising? Will people notice if I put on five pounds? Will that slice of my son's birthday cake make me look fat?"

For many individuals, their life can be held hostage by the terror of weight gain. Overwhelmingly, messages about eating, exercise, the scale, and what people think about them are characteristic of an eating disorder. Eating disordered thoughts sabotage quality of life.

Quality of life is a particularly significant issue of interest for many individuals. As a result, researchers often administer questionnaires (QOLQ) to collect relevant information on this factor. Questions about energy for school or work, overall health, social and family relationships, and life satisfaction overall are typically included in a quality of life questionnaire. The same survey is often given to patients with chronic illnesses in an effort to understand the effects of illness on their overall health and functioning.

Results have consistently demonstrated that people who struggle with morbid obesity have a lower quality of life than people with other mental illness and people with cancer. They feel isolated, sad, and judged. They sometimes experience self-hatred. In reality, some individuals who are desperate to change are driven to the operating table. According to one study, individuals who were obese sought surgical treatment because of their interest in an improved quality of life.

The biting reality is that while the hypothetically "perfectly thin" might be considered a success by culture, individuals of any size or weight might feel just as sad, lost, and betrayed by the culture as the morbidly obese. The extremes of cultural weight success or failure may lead to emotional frustration for many individuals. Figure 3-2 illustrates the cultural cycle of weight failure.

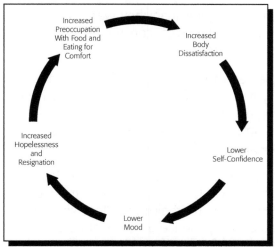

Figure 3-2. The cultural cycle of weight failure

It is difficult for most individuals to imagine that their weight is not fundamentally related to happiness. The culture equates happiness with perfect weight and perfect performance in so many areas of life, including academics, sports, music, and material possessions, etc. "Race to Nowhere" is a documentary that delves into the lives of America's students and captures the brokenness of the perfect-is-everything culture. Students, experts, and statistics narrate heartbreaking story after heartbreaking story of how the pull to perfection leads to stress, anxiety, depression, addiction, cutting, eating disorders, and even suicide. While the film was created to prompt awareness of and improvement in America's education system, the overarching message of, "our students are pressured to perform but are failing," resonates with those individuals who work with individuals who are frustrated with their weight.

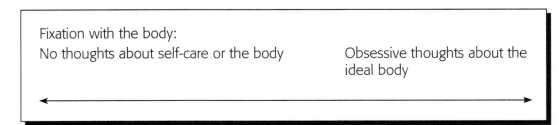

Fixation with the body:
No thoughts about self-care or the body   Obsessive thoughts about the ideal body

What if "perfection" was not the only measure of success? A YouTube video that went viral in 2013 showed the response of a father to his son's exclamation that he had just received a "C" on a math text. The tearful celebration of the father for his son's achievement was moving. A friend's son, who is particularly good at math, saw the video and said, "It's only a C." His reaction was similar to those individuals who see only the "fat," without understanding the greater context. They may see 'size', without understanding the genetics. They may see 'shape,' without appreciating their weight history and related factors. They may see 'fat," but don't see the "person." The weight may be actually 30 pounds lighter than they were just a year earlier. Weight change may be the result of healthy eating (e.g., consuming more vegetables), a drug problem, or a devastating illness. In the words of Picasso, "They look but do not see."

Commonly, people tend to discount another individual's progress in a particular undertaking, especially if the belief, task, or goal is perceived as easy to achieve. For example, if maintaining a stable and low weight has always been simple for you, then you likely believe it is simple for others as well. You might conclude that maintaining an ideal weight is a snap.

But, what if success is unique to each individual? What if success is more than a number? What if success isn't always skinny? What if a student or mom or executive doesn't have to wait until they hit their pre-college dress or suit size to be and feel successful? Is it possible to experience a sense of accomplishment in the process of everyday life—every single day? *What if success were framed differently?*

Over three decades ago, when the obesity rate hovered at 12 percent, but was on the rise, clinical psychologist and researcher, Peter M. Miller, wrote an article, "Redefining Success in Eating Disorders," a commentary that has gone largely unnoticed by the throngs of pundits, scholars, doctors, and educators trying to crack the code on obesity. While recognizing the complexity of eating disorders, including obesity, Miller asked, "Do we know what we should be measuring in the first place?" In his article, he challenged the narrow definitions of weight success, including those that rely on the dichotomous thinking perpetuated by the over-idealization of thin and reliance on BMI scores. His most provocative call-to-arms was the following:

> Clinicians must begin to view outcome as a continuous process rather than a definitive end product. Outcome measures must take into account a multifaceted, psychobiological model of eating disorders in which continuous care with stages of success is the norm. Various outcomes must be considered including the overall physical and psychological health of the patient regardless of absolute changes in weight or bingeing.

In reality, Miller was ahead of his time. He advocated for more moderate weight-related goals; for recognition of improved health with modest weight change; for a focus on process, rather than only outcome; and, for consideration of psychosocial variables in defining success. If only the world had listened to him, given that statistics show that the culture-wide diet obsession has not curbed obesity. In a little over two decades, American obesity has risen from 12.3 percent (1990) to 35.7 percent (2015).

Miller's thoughts also apply to exercise programs. From the standpoint of good health, the process of being active is more important than the product of reaching an ideal endpoint. Fitness, like body weight, is influenced by genetics, while activity is a behavior that is affected more by the environment. Because of their genetic background, some people will never reach ideal fit or thin, but they can be healthier, if they lead a physically active life. The point is reinforced by renowned researchers Rod Dishman, Gregory Heath, and I-Min Lee in their book, *Physical Activity Epidemiology*, who wrote "A change from preoccupation with scale weight to healthful management of blood pressure, blood glucose, and blood lipid levels through prudent diet and regular physical activity in pursuit of moderate fitness, is perhaps a more important health goal for most people".

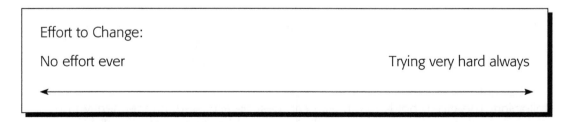

Effort to Change:

No effort ever   Trying very hard always

American culture holds that overweight people just aren't working hard enough to exercise and lose the weight. As such, Nike's "Just Do It!" campaign permeates the cultural psyche of Americans 25 years after its launch. At a recent lunch with an investment banker, a friend brought up the topic of weight loss, after he noticed his colleague in the financial services industry looked as if he had lost a few pounds. "It's simple," the man responded. "I just eat less. I had a friend who lost 25 pounds by simply eating only half of the portions he received at restaurants. If he went to McDonald's, he'd just eat half his fries and half his Big Mac."

Good for him. On the other hand, this approach might not be a "simple" and successful strategy for everyone. For example, some people may find it difficult to adhere to this kind of portion control. Others might have difficulty sustaining such a strategy over a longer course of time. Still others might feel deprived or punished by this degree of caloric restriction.

Some individuals may have difficulty losing weight without engaging in increased amounts of exercise. It should be noted, however, that equal levels of caloric restriction or comparable amounts of physical activity will not result in equal weight loss for all people. In order for a weight loss strategy to be successful, it must suit the unique needs, interests, and attributes of the individual involved. Some individuals may not like restaurant eating at all and would prefer to avoid strategies requiring eating in restaurants. Others may like to eat out.

Successfully managing weight is often a pathway strewn with obstacles. One such obstacle, often is extensive amounts of negative self-talk, which sabotage healthy efforts. What if family and friends become competitive or have hostile feelings about noticing weight loss among others? What if they have larger amounts of food to help cope with their emotions and subsequently feel unable to manage their stress? What if they tried to "just do it" before, but failed? The presupposition is that if they can't "just do it," then they are a failure. Next time, dig in and try harder, right?

Wrong. It's not always a matter of just working harder.

CHANGE IN WORLDVIEW

A new and positive future for weight managment requires a change in perspective. In some ways, such a model is conceptual, before it is practical. It is seeing the world differently. One alternative view of weight loss comes from a grassroots movement that subsequently became Health at Every Size (HAES). The group originated in the 1960s, with the publication of the provocative article, "More People Should Be Fat!"

Currently, the HAES organization, led by Linda Bacon, PhD., has a substantial following. The group holds that health can best be achieved independently from size. The movement supports people—of all sizes—in addressing health directly via adopting healthy behaviors. It is built on the following tenets:
• Accepting and respecting the natural diversity of body sizes and shapes

- Eating in a flexible manner that values pleasure and honors internal cues of hunger, satiety, and appetite
- Finding the joy in moving one's body and becoming more physically vital

The awareness that the HAES organization creates regarding health and dieting is encouraging. "Accepting the body and shape that you have" is a useful suggestion, especially since it will be the only body you ever will have and that considerable literature suggests that changes in weight or shape do no always bring improved body satisfaction. A risk exists, however, that acceptance may also be interpreted by the masses as "I don't have to do anything to take care of myself." The dust jacket of Bacon's book Health at Every Size: The Surprising Truth about Your Weight echoes a similar ethos: "Read it, and you may be convinced that the best way to win the war against fat is to give up the fight."

While such a strategy could work for some individuals, it may not be the best fit for all. The obese condition is not one condition. Weight status is the outward manifestation of many conditions. One approach will likely not suit all people or conditions. What *UnWeighted Nation* is proposing is an exit from the diet or don't diet thinking. What this book is advancing is an end to this "either-or" debate.

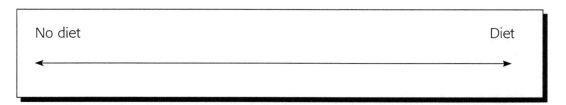

Instead, the *"UnWeighted"* model encourages the consideration of the diet versus no-diet debate along a continuum of possibilities: On one end of the continuum is "diet," while on the opposite and extreme end is "no-diet." The primary focus of the "diet" camp is an outcome-orientation, organized around caloric restriction and pounds lost. Historically, diets were motivated by appearance and/or health, and were always organized around the number of pounds lost.

In contrast, at the other end of the continuum, is a "no-diet approach." The no-diet approach is not outcome-focused, does not advise caloric restriction, and does not target weight loss. Theoretically speaking, at the most extreme end of a no-diet approach is permission to *stop* thinking about food choices, calories, exercise, appearance, weight loss, and health matters altogether.

The *"UnWeighted"* model invites individuals to choose strategies located between the two poles on the "diet-no-diet continuum" that depict the focus, behavior, belief, and effort that they feel are appropriate for them. This choice permits flexibility and change in decision-making over a individual's lifetime. Success is then defined uniquely for each specific person and should be accepted and respected by others. This approach invites the consideration of strategies found anywhere on the spectrum of possibilities.

The *"UnWeighted"* model permits change of perspective and behavior over time. This approach is a step away from the dieting-no dieting debate and instead organizes effort around each person's individual preferences and values: health interests, needs, allocation of time and energy, available resources, etc. Importantly, these values are grounded within each individual and, as much, are oriented to personal choices, rather than more external dictates. The model recognizes that humans, behavior and intentions are imperfect, while better health can be attained despite these imperfections.

Because this model reduces the burdensome focus on weight-loss, the approach is deemed the *"UnWeighted"* model. This model allows health-related decisions to be considered along a continuum. The model encourages individuals to embrace self-care; focus more on the process; focus less on the outcome; develop greater internal control; foster emotional awareness; engage in positive self-talk; and enable an individual to compare their success more with their own personally established goals, and less to a universal externally derived standards.

An *"UnWeighted"* healthcare plan does not promise "an ideal body" or "ideal health." It does, however, promise better health and better well-being. It should be noted that the model may not please a person's physician, who may still be focused on reducing BMI. On the other hand, by navigating a reasonable middle ground between the two opposite polarities of dieting and non-dieting, better health, better control of mind and body, and greater confidence can be achieved.

The underlying premise of the *"UnWeighted"* approach is that success is not about being skinny or losing every pound, or looking like someone on the cover of *Vogue*. As such, efforts and expectations to do so will cause more harm than good. In contrast, success in this model is learning and growing into a healthier you over your lifetime.

Successful self-care allows freedom to focus on the present, rather than obsessing about a future that is so remote that an individual's motivation to focus on today is lost altogether. Life-long self-care is a process. It's not an all-or-nothing undertaking. Inner strength and confidence are developed in small, successful, daily decisions that empower a person. For example, "Today, I want to go for a walk, eat more vegetables, and spend time with good friends. I give myself permission to plan differently for tomorrow."

Typically, diets are highly restrictive, challenging the individual to eat as little as possible in order to lose as much weight as possible. Alternatively, the no-diet approach means, "I can eat whatever I want, with no restrictions." In comparison, the *"UnWeighted"* plan says, "Look for a balance and navigate the challenges that seem right for you." With the dieting approach, the frequency of eating is determined by the rules of the diet plan. A no-dieting approach, in contrast, does not require focusing on eating frequency, portion size, ingredients, or content, etc.

Traditional dieting is fueled by "black-and-white" thinking. Either you're on the diet, or you are off of it. In a traditional diet, you're bad and feel guilty if you eat a thousand calories of chips and queso at the neighborhood block party and you are viewed as "good" if you are able to say "no."

The approach advocated in this book prescribes a different perspective. In a traditional diet, the reward is external, e.g., people clapping for pounds lost at a meeting, a bonus for reaching weight-loss goals at the office, the reward you promised yourself (i.e., the new outfit, fishing rod, or vacation), and dollars offered toward the cost of a health insurance plan, etc.

In the proposed healthier *"UnWeighted"* approach, the rewards are more likely to be internal in nature, with less pressure, greater self-efficacy, more acceptable expectations, a sustained degree of confidence, and a growing level of self-esteem. With an *"UnWeighted"* plan, it is okay to change what you eat day to day. People change, goals change, and life conditions change. One week, you may be on a cruise, surrounded by buffet dining. One day, you may be in Belgium and want a Belgian waffle. And so, you have one. Furthermore, if you are in Belgium on a business trip, you may miss a couple days of exercise. That's okay too.

In the *"UnWeighted"* model, you are encouraged to observe your behavior and be fully aware of the health risks and responsibilities of your actions. Also in accordance with this model, one avoids self-recrimination and punishment for making less-than-optimal choices. You are encouraged to be challenged, to learn, to apply what you learn, and make decisions that feel right for you.

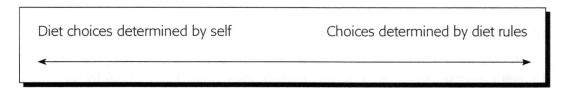

Diet choices determined by self   Choices determined by diet rules

EMOTIONAL AWARENESS

The traditional approach to dieting fails more often than not. One reason for the high rates of relapse may for some individuals be emotional factors.

Many individuals may not completely understand weight gain following weight loss. They may not realize how they arrived at their current weight. What caused them to gain so much weight? What's behind their eating at 9:30 each night? Why the obsession with their weight? What are their feelings about health in general? What triggers the desire for Ben and Jerry's, when everything inside them screams, "You'll regret it in 15 minutes"? While eating behavior and weight may be about genetics, culture, biology, hunger and more, it might also be influenced by internal emotional states.

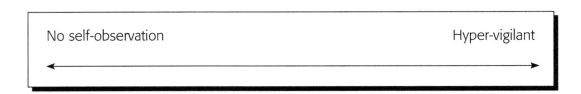

No self-observation   Hyper-vigilant

At the heart of the *"UnWeighted"* model is the assumption that it is helpful to understand who you are and what you really want, as well as how the outside world is affecting you. A big chunk of emotional awareness is rooted in healthy relationships. In more traditional dieting, focusing on relationships is not always a priority.

In the *"UnWeighted"* model, close and supportive relationships are deemed as central and vital to good health. Without healthy relationships in place, a relationship with food may be an imperfect substitute.

In the *"UnWeighted"* model, the whole person is considered. Individuals are asked about their interests and motivations in general. For example, "You want to lose weight. What do you believe the weight loss will provide you and other than weight loss, what else are you wanting for yourself?" The question sometimes gives pause to silence.

So many individuals have been so focused on their weight that little else seems to matter. There is often the sense that all other life interests and passion will be found after the weight loss is realized. Over time, individuals are able to identify non-weight related wishes, needs, and desires. With 50 individuals, there will often be 50 different responses. One gentleman may want an improved level of energy. Another might simply may want to be able to walk down the aisle at his daughter's wedding. Yet another person want to be able to ski with his kids in his 50s and 60s, while another might want to feel better about themselves.

The proposed "UnWeighted" model is not a steel-framed approach; it's fluid. Different people at different times in their lives have different preferences and interests. Each will have different goals and a unique path in reaching their goals. The *"UnWeighted"* model is not a one-size-fits-all fix. Even more importantly, it is not a "fix." In reality, the *"UnWeighted"* model is a "process."

An acquaintance shared the story of how she experienced a shift to using this healthier model. She grew tired of obsessing about how many days she exercised a week, as well as what to eat and how much to eat, while waiting for the numbers on the scale to tell her if her efforts had been good enough. Her search for the lowest-calorie protein bar and the largest diet soda was both endless and fatiguing.

She would not be labeled hugely overweight by most observers. Admittedly, however, she relentlessly pursued being thin. She had read the magazines and heard the talk shows. Intellectually, she worked hard to force herself to believe that "size ultimately didn't matter."

On the other hand, when she let go of the obsessing, she put on 12 pounds in two months. She felt angry and out of control. She felt like both science and her body had once again deceived her. In response, she reverted to a "non-dieting approach." The resultant free-for-all was absent of mindfulness. She tossed out all rules and restrictions. She felt out of control, and the pounds quickly found their new home.

Identifying the "polar extremes" is easier than finding the safe middle. Finding the right balance of challenge and comfort can take time. It requires trial and error, and, as they say, tweaking. A good indicator that you may not be living in the more balanced survivable middle is the sense of feeling emotionally over-controlled or out of control, which is what she experienced when she tried not to care.

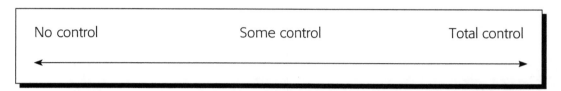

In failing, however, she learned more about a strategy that felt right for her. This new sense of reality meant letting go of the "lose-it-all-forever dream," as well as the incessant obsessions that went with that. On the other hand, living more in the middle of the continuum of possibilities is a choice she could learn to accept and appreciate. It was not consistent with the messages she had been surrounded by forever. It required letting go of the more ideal frame she had clipped out of the magazine and posted on the door of her refrigerator. She had so often envisioned that ideal frame being her frame.

Pursuing the more modest goals were components of a lifestyle that she could imagine doing for a lifetime. She could imagine a doable path to improved health. Her path.

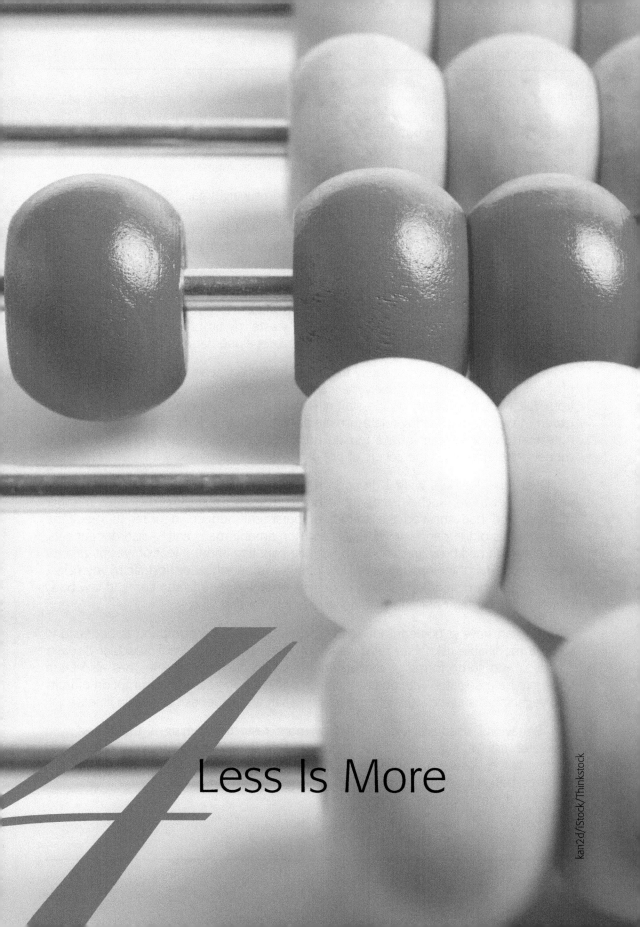

4 Less Is More

Fifteen grapes, a carefully measured half-slice of unbuttered whole wheat toast, a quarter cup of nonfat cottage cheese, and a liter of water—such was her morning diet. There would be nothing but water for the rest of the day and nothing during her daily five to six hours of dance and conditioning. Dinner was the same routine each night: two ounces of skinless chicken breast and a handful of vegetables.

Like most ballet dancers, Rachel was terrified of weight gain. She knew the dance attire would betray any sweet, salty, or fatty indulgence. Her physique was scrutinized as sharply as her form. In response, she starved and plié-ed her way toward what she believed to be her instructor's expectations for the "perfect figure." Any noticeable added ounces risked her being hit with the cane, leaving red and blue welts for days.

Even worse, she chanced being reprimanded in front of the class: "Apparently you don't want to be a dancer anymore." "Did you decide to give up?" "Did you want to dance today or just hang around and eat and waste my time?" Or, "I'm surprised you have enough energy to get that body out of bed, let alone dance."

A perfect figure, however, rarely translates to perfect health, whether emotional or physical. The body is "not infinitely malleable," says Kelly Brownell, formerly a professor from Yale, who is currently on the staff at Duke University, as well as a highly regarded expert in weight- and eating-related matters. With regard to Rachael, it is important to note that only 2 percent of the female population might naturally be as thin as the models who appear on the covers of popular fashion magazines.

Over time, Rachel's weight dropped to a dangerous 90 pounds during her dance years. To get there, Rachel lived with a highly rigid and restrictive diet for a number of years and had survived the torture of persistent hunger, in order to meet the requirements of the dance world. As is common among many eating-disorder patients, Rachel's mind had been imprisoned by calorie counting and the fear of weight gain for many years. Hair thinning, bad acne, low energy, amenorrhea, orthostatic hypotension, or dizziness when standing (all consequences of prolonged malnutrition and low-body weight) did not deter her efforts to achieve being "thin" at all costs.

Diet can have a powerful influence on health. Food consumption is understood to be a modifiable risk factor for a variety of illnesses, such as cardiovascular disease, diabetes, and some forms of cancer. Adherence to dietary guidelines has also been shown to be associated with better health. In particular, increased consumption of fruits and vegetables is associated with improved health and lower risk of certain illnesses.

Behavioral scientists know well that more restrictive dieting is associated with a greater risk of subsequent overeating and/or binge eating. Dieting, stress, and intermittent exposure to foods with high sugar content may also increase the risk of binge behavior. A history of addiction in genetically related family members also increases the risk of binge eating.

Predictably, Rachel's dance pursuits eventually came to an end, and her pattern of restrictive eating was soon replaced by out-of-control binge eating. Her weight escalated to well over 200 pounds. The added pounds were accompanied by the barrage of "fat feelings," self-hate, and recrimination. Hers was not the body she knew, not the body she believed men wanted to date, and not the body that culture typically declared beautiful.

After months of counseling, Rachel reluctantly agreed to resist the urges to "lose all the weight" and to embrace a manageable weight at 149 pounds, 75 pounds less than her highest weight. On her five-foot-four-inch frame, this weight was far from her ballerina-best. On the other hand, it was better for her.

It seemed to be a weight that could be sustained, given her lifestyle, age, and health status. It was a weight that her body permitted with some (but not intense) attention to regular exercise and some attention to healthy eating. Rachel began to grasp that when her weight dropped beneath 149 pounds, her anorexia reawakened. Below 149, nothing became more important than peeling away just one more pound. Obsessive and compulsive thoughts returned with a vengeance. Self-loathing and a pursuit of perfection took over her thoughts.

When in therapy, she considered, "What do I want for myself and my health?" Was there more to life than weighing in at the "perfect" 120-pound college weight? In time, she understood that the weight-related numbers obsession, although troubling, offered her relief from other more distressing thoughts.

It took some time before Rachel could imagine anything more satisfying than the perfect weight. It also took time to talk about the "more distressing thoughts" and to learn other strategies for coping. Gradually, her newfound success felt more satisfying than the relentless pursuit of thin.

Years later at work, the health insurance company requested a health evaluation for all employees at her worksite. She answered "no" to questions about smoking and drinking alcohol in excess. She answered "yes" to driving with a seat belt, yearly doctor visits, twice yearly dental appointments, and regular exercise, etc. In addition, body weight was measured, body composition was assessed, and BMI calculated.

The numbers, which reflected scrutiny and the evaluation process in general, renewed previous worries about her body, weight, and fat. Her lab results were highlighted in blue, indicating "within a healthy range." Her weight and BMI were highlighted in red. The insurance company put her on alert for higher premiums, since her body weight fell in the "overweight" category, and her BMI landed in the "above normal" range. Compared with national population norms for women of her age, she was considered to be of lower weight than most. Nonetheless, the insurance company concluded that she was a "health risk."

"See, even my insurance company says I'm too fat," she said. "I think I should lose more weight." "Because the insurance company says so?" she was asked. "They can look at a chart and see that the numbers are not within 'ideal' norms. On the other hand, does that accurately and completely describe who you are or your history? Does the chart know and does the insurance company know what is best for your health?"

When the insurance company documented her overweight status in red, it created panic. Yes, her weight was outside an ideal range, according to a "chart." A lower weight would mean less red writing on her report, but it would also mean the re-emergence of an eating disorder and its associated depression, low self-esteem, anxiety, isolation, and obsessive thinking. The insurance company did not know that she ate healthy meals, containing foods from all food groups appropriately throughout the day; that she exercised regularly; and that she was no longer refusing to see doctors because of fear of being weighed. Furthermore, they did not know that a stable weight for her was healthier than the repeated weight gain and weight-loss cycles, and the emotional torture of starvation. Simply stated, the insurance company did not know what was best for her.

YOUR BEST YOU

Do you know what is best for you? It's a question that many individuals don't pause to ask. When it comes to weight, Americans commonly believe thin is best, accentuated by six-pack abdominals, cut biceps, inner thigh gaps, hollow cheeks, and pencil thin arms. As such, the promise of power, reward, and acceptance is sufficient to cause the masses to blindly pursue the deity of thin. Even if dieting has caused a cycle of weight loss and weight gain; even if gastric bypass surgery has led to bowel obstructions, dumping syndrome, or alcohol addiction; even if obsession with the thin ideal has led to depression, anxiety, eating disorders, self-hatred, and alienation—the culture still believes that thin is best. As a result, individuals continue to pursue thin with zeal. They exert themselves on cardio. Lift more weights. Cut out sugars and carbs. Count points. Take some pills. Sign on for surgical change. Eventually, however, they flog themselves when they haven't arrived.

It's hard not to be seduced by the promises of the thin and its evil twin sister, the diet mentality. Who wouldn't buy the promise of more money, more friends, more power, and more beauty? A quick fix to a perfect body, after a lifetime of weight struggle, is a siren song. Drill down on the number, follow the plan, and sweat it out is the promised path to life satisfaction.

Too many people, however, feel stuck in the land of "not-good-enough." For these individuals, it is not about "wanting" to lose weight; it is feeling they "must" lost weight—at all costs. They don't completely understand *why* this situation is so. Furthermore, they might not know what any other success might look like for them. Separate from the pursuit of the "thin ideal," does some sense of other personal identity exist for them?

Just as much as the body, the mind must be engaged in any weight-related journey. In reality, personal reflection can help uncover factors that have led to weight stagnation, escalation, or cycling. A lot can be learned from noticing patterns related to weight and eating-related history, especially when the person's corresponding social and emotional history are examined.

Accordingly, individuals might notice cycles of gain, loss, and more gain. Perhaps more importantly, they may recall a time when they briefly were at their lowest weight, and at that weight, they were not always their happiest or healthiest self. Many individuals may recite a litany of failed diets and extreme periods of deprivation. For example, there is the 22-hour-fasting diet, and there is the two-hour-eat-anything-you-want diet. There is also the "eat only grapefruit diet" and the "eat only meat diet". All these diets are time-limited. Because they all cannot be sustained and eventually end. Unfortunately, the frustration and sense of failure continues. Some remember how diet-burnout led them to adopt a "screw-it" approach to health—eat anything, in any amount, and at any time.

It is important to note that eating and mood are reciprocally related. Problematic eating can influence emotion, and negative emotion can influence eating and attitudes about body shape and size. It can be beneficial for individuals to notice and learn from these patterns.

Some individuals describe the incessant talk in their head offering minute-by-minute critique: "Don't eat that. You don't deserve that. That food is bad for you. You are such a pig. You know you can't control yourself. That will make you fat! You are weak!" Eventually, many dieters consign themselves to the curtain-closing resignation on their efforts: "I can't do it! I give up."

A client was completing a questionnaire with 20 to 30 questions about eating, diet, and mood. There was a blank space of approximately two inches allotted for examples of messages an individual might "hear in their head" about food, eating, and body. The client answered the question using that space and then flipped the page over to the blank side and filled every bit of space with an endless list of critical, negative and hurtful words. For this person, as it does for many people, the fear of fat supersedes all else.

The bigger questions are: Are you content? Are you able to do what's important to you in life? Aside from your weight, is your health what you want it to be? Do you want to be doing anything differently and why? What makes it hard to do more of what you prefer to be doing? What would success look like for you? Is your description of success your own or what someone else wants for you? What are your motivations to change or improve the way you take care of yourself? How do you understand your motivation to change or not change?

The chronic "dieter's life" can be a roller coaster of emotional and physical change—brief and fleeting sugary highs, mixed with dark, heavy, indulgent lows. More diet attempts are an indication of likely poor dieting adherence. The search can feel endless and increasingly hopeless. As time passes, the rollercoaster zaps energy and personal confidence.

Many individuals cannot imagine what success beyond their desired weight might look like. Some have big dreams, but are crushed by the memories of past failure. Some fear what change will entail. After all, big change can mean extensive public scrutiny and greater potential for humiliation, if things subsequently slide out of control.

Exiled in the land of self-defeat, a healthy-self is a foreign-self. That situation is partly because "healthy" in our culture is often defined by the standards of the culture, rather than by the unique circumstances of each individual. Individuals struggle, at times, to know themselves through their own lens, opposed to solely through society's lens. When clients are asked to discuss how they define success, what they value, what provides them satisfaction, what they want for their health or body, many individuals struggle to have answers that are uniquely theirs and not just the repeated version of what they have heard others say all around them during the course of their lives.

When asked how she takes care of herself after a stressful day, the highly intelligent 50-year-old, with an accomplished medical career, looked back blankly. The answers that followed were, "Uh … read a book." "Uh … get a manicure." "Uh… (and laughing with a little embarrassment) I don't know. What am I supposed to say?"

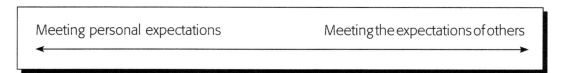

As a rule, most individuals are oriented to the "shoulds" and the "suppose—to's." In time, they may become more oriented to the expectations of teachers, parents, boss, spouse, or friends, and less aware of the personal values and wishes that emerge from within themselves. They know what is required to achieve the As, get the raise at work, or please a spouse. They know what their friends want and expect and when these colleagues will or will not be forgiving. While they are keenly attuned to the needs of others, they are less so to their own needs.

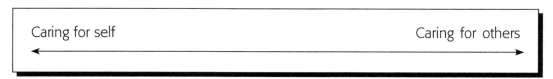

"I imagine you know in detail how your mother, father, husband, and children take care of themselves emotionally," her therapist said. "It sounds like you know more about *their* emotional needs than your own."

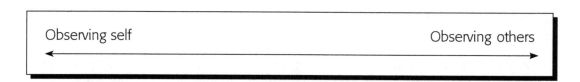

| Observing self | Observing others |

Better understanding their own emotional needs is an important step in being able to make better informed, healthy decisions about body and eating behavior.

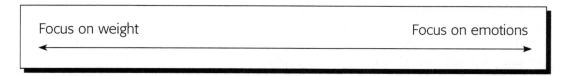

| Focus on weight | Focus on emotions |

ADVERSE CONSEQUENCES

Setting goals that are focused on any extreme, such as a large weight loss, a torturous exercise regimen, or a highly restrictive eating, is a set-up to failure. Many participants become frustrated with their slow progress. Other individuals struggle to adhere to eating and exercise regimens that feel punishing. Some people come to believe that their long-term health benefits are not worth the immediate time and effort required. Drop-out rates for individuals engaged in intensive "weight loss" programs are high, especially in the first three to six months of a program. Some attrition rates in weight-loss programs are as high as 60 percent.

High attrition is disappointing, but predictable, since compliance rates in many healthcare arenas are traditionally poor. For example, only 25 percent of individuals with chronic illness use medications as prescribed, resulting in morbidity- and mortality-related costs, estimated to be 100 billion. Even when the benefits of healthcare guidelines are well documented, compliance is often poor. For example, appropriate and regular use of blood pressure medication has a documented benefit in reducing the risk of several health-related conditions and illnesses, such as stroke, myocardial infarction, hospitalization, and patient mortality. Adherence rates to taking this medication, however, are roughly 50 percent. Even among highly-trained medical personnel working in hospitals, researchers found a 51 percent compliance rate for hand-hygiene protocols, with physicians having a lower compliance than nurses.

Factors associated with poor adherence "are multilevel and relate not only to the patient, but also to the provider, healthcare system, healthcare organization and the community." Adherence rates for dieting and exercise programs are similarly poor.

More often than not, diet success is a reflection of the numbers on the scale. Highly respected in the industry, physical fitness and epidemiology researchers Rod Dishman, Gregory Heath, and I-Min Lee propose shifting the focus away from the numbers and toward health-related factors, such as blood pressure, blood glucose, blood lipid levels, moderate physical activity, and healthy eating.

A shift away from numbers is vital. In fact, the literature on motivation to change behavior for the purpose of improving health shows that health is not improved by numbers alone. As is known, knowledge is not always followed by action (e.g., smoking). An awareness of the benefits of exercise and healthy eating is not always sufficient to motivate improved self-care.

A number of factors can impede health practice-related adherence, including low motivation, insufficient time, fatigue, inconvenience, poor access to facilities, boredom, and limiting health factors (e.g., age, illness, or injury). Low self-esteem and depression are also inversely related to positive health practices. However other factors can improve compliance, such as age, education, and socio-economic status. Goal setting, self-monitoring, and self-reward can also improve adherence, as can internal locus of control, self-confidence, and inner strength. These qualities collectively serve as the core of healthy self-care.

Successful self-care means finding the balance between an obsessive focus on diet, weight, and exercise, and the complete abandonment of health. Living in either extreme is problematic. Living in the "I don't care" mode can leave you feeling out of control and making excuses to stay that way. Living in the hyperfocused diet mode can be punishing, depriving, and exhausting. Both extremes result in the individual feeling the brunt of failure.

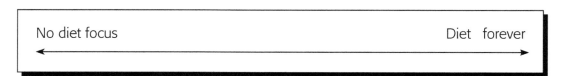

Historically, eating disorders have been difficult to treat, especially for individuals who have longer-term illness. A study conducted at the University of Sydney studied how different kinds of treatment benefitted individuals with chronic eating disorders for an average of 15 years. Results showed that treatments focused predominantly on numbers were far less successful than treatments that were oriented to individual patient values. When individuals focus less on perfection and more on what they value, they find more life satisfaction and better health. Brené Brown, a renowned author who received attention after her TED talk on the power of vulnerability, makes the fine distinction between striving for perfection and striving for excellence. She writes:

> *Perfectionism is not the same thing as striving for excellence. Perfectionism is not about healthy achievement and growth. Perfectionism is a 20-ton shield that we lug around, thinking it will protect us, when, in fact, it's the thing that's really preventing us from being seen.*

Perfectionism is not self-improvement. Perfectionism is, at its core, about trying to earn approval. Most perfectionists grew up being praised for achievement and performance (grades, manners, rule following, people pleasing, appearance, sports).

Somewhere along the way, they adopted this dangerous and debilitating belief system: "I am what I accomplish and how well I accomplish it. Please. Perform. Perfect." Healthy striving is self-focused: How can I improve? Perfectionism is other-focused: What will they think? Perfectionism is a hustle.

Lugging around the "20-ton shield" of perfection can be exhausting. Deep in our sense of self is the cultural lie that tells us that physical perfection makes us worthy, just like our physical imperfections make us unworthy. No amount of weight loss can mend the gap between our perceived external worth and actual internal worth. It is in the hustle of pleasing and performing that individuals miss the opportunity to satisfy their internal longings, what they really want, and what gives them joy. What if those individuals who struggled with their weight reframed success as achieving overall better health and well-being rather than "being the best"?

A local college soccer team at a small liberal arts college got a shot at playing the nation's top ranked team in their division. Top dog and underdog battled it out. Ultimately, our local team lost by one goal. When asked about the game, the players agreed, "It was the best game we ever played!" While they admitted disappointment, they were exhilarated and proud. This team didn't have the winning score, but their focus, attitude, appreciation of their talent, effort, and collaboration on the field was the stuff that makes champions. The score or number alone didn't tell the whole story. This team didn't score the most goals, but it was their best play.

It is important to be aware that what is best for you may not be what others— or culture—think is best. Numerous sources report that a simple weight reduction of 10 percent of the total body weight is significantly associated with reduction of high blood pressure, a decrease in high levels of cholesterol, and a diminished risk of sudden death. Even a five percent weight loss has been shown to produce medically measurable results.

Health benefits occur long before reaching an ultimately lower weight. When weight loss does not translate to "perfect" numbers, feelings of failure can erupt. When that situation arises, inner voices cry, "Not good enough." Yet, the resultant weight might be reasonable for that particular person. In reality, a "best weight" for a person is one less determined by numbers and more by "maintainability," amidst a lifestyle that is satisfying.

For a person steeped in the diet culture, it is often difficult to reconcile that a less rigid approach to weight loss might actually produce better results than would an all-or-nothing approach. Unfortunately, this method is not the approach that advertisers sell.

Healthy adults are able to observe themselves, and know themselves, as well as understand why some strategies are best for them. Traditional dieting pushes its followers to unsustainable extremes. The rules of dieting tend to feel confining and restrictive, which often leads to anxiety and a decreased level of satisfaction of life. On the other hand, a dieting approach without rules feels chaotic, often causing the dieter to give up.

In contrast, self-directed guidelines are freeing. Individuals who develop their own self-care plan are free to learn what works or doesn't work for them, make adjustments in their goals and behaviors at any time, and, ultimately, maintain control over their self-care options. The right of an individual to choose and the freedom to change their choices can feel adult-like, liberating, and independent.

ONGOING AND OBJECTIVE SELF-REFLECTION

Jessica was a young adult whose weight bounced up and down. She felt out of control and guilty for not being able to control her weight. Her parents were teased and bullied about their weight and believed "fat" was unattractive. Each parent had lost a parent to cardiovascular disease at an early age.

They feared that their daughter could not control herself enough to avoid unwanted weight gain. Because her parents worried about her health and well-being, they instituted an array of eating restrictions for her. No sweets. No soda. No chips. No processed food. No fast food. No eating after 6 p.m.

When they noticed Jessica eating unapproved items, they scolded her and locked up the snacks. Their response made Jessica feel weak and bad. Unfortunately, however, their reactions only intensified Jessica's desire for the forbidden foods. Gradually, Jessica's weight crept up. Under the guise of night, Jessica would sneak slices of bread. One slice out of a 20-slice loaf went undetected. If unseen, she told herself, there would be no shame. The situation, however, hounded her into adulthood.

As an adult, Jessica inhaled her food. Her brain couldn't catch up with her stomach to say, "Slow down!" or "Stop!" Overeating led to weight gain. When asked about her speed-eating, she said she felt guilty when she ate. She often still feared judgment, even though her parents lived miles away. The message she continued to tell herself was, "Eat quickly, before I am discovered, and the food is taken away." Speed-eating in that moment was an escape from the shame of the eating experience itself. While she shielded herself from the emotional discomfort, she lost control of her health.

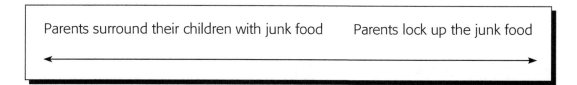

Parents surround their children with junk food　　　Parents lock up the junk food

When she intentionally slowed down the pace of her eating, for the first time, she noticed gradations of fullness. In slowing down, she worked hard to remind herself that she need not feel guilty; that being punished for eating was about her past and not her future; that eating was not a criminal act; that she wouldn't get in trouble; and that she was an adult who owned her choices.

As a result of slowing down her eating and challenging the old patterns of automatic thoughts and feelings, she discovered the details of taste and texture not previously known. The Styrofoam texture of baked potato chips and the chalkiness of no-fat yogurt, two staples of her low-fat diet, bothered her. She said, "Now, I eat the real thing, which I love. When I eat slowly, I feel more satisfied with the flavor of what I am eating and don't feel like I always have to eat it all."

Jessica's observations allowed her to discover what foods satisfied her, to monitor how full she was feeling, and to acknowledge the control she had over her life. She experienced the freedom of choice, as well as freedom from old messages.

The "more" middle ground of weight success demands ongoing and objective self-observation. As such, individuals need to be aware of their emotions, as well as well as their thoughts and beliefs about what is important. Such an awareness is the cornerstone of healthy eating.

Each person is positioned in a constant state of learning and refining. When their weight plateaus or creeps back up, a person has the opportunity to notice the situation, and then learn and apply this information to their subsequent decision-making. Do they have reasonable expectations? Are they continuing to pursue health and self-care? Is their internal dialogue void of criticism? Do they have an adjusted plan of action that feels right for them and is their choice?

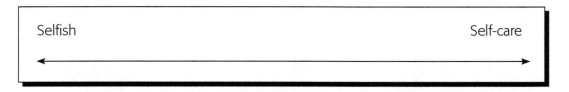

Selfish　　　　　　　　　　　　　　　　　　　　　　　　　　　Self-care

INNER CHOICES

Good health depends on *mindfulness*. Mindfulness is currently in vogue in many psychology circles. In general, mindfulness is the ability to be self-aware and completely present with yourself in any given moment. A researcher on mindfulness, Jon Kabat-Zin, described the attribute this way: "The awareness that emerges through paying attention on purpose, in the present moment, and nonjudgmentally to the unfolding of experience moment by moment."

Throughout the world, for thousands of years, mindfulness and meditation have been taught and practiced in various religions, such as Islam, Buddhism, Christianity, and Judaism. More recently, mindfulness has become a fundamental component of psychotherapy practice for various conditions, including pain, depression, anxiety, and binge eating.

Mindfulness training and practice are fundamental to "dialectic behavior therapy." This form of treatment is effective in supporting healthy self-regulation, as well as healthy eating and self-care.

Mindfulness is a precursor of change and growth, and what humanistic psychologists called "self-actualization." Defined as the full realization of an individual's potential, the theory posits that what a human requires in order to grow already exists within each person. Abraham Maslow, a leading thinker of the humanistic movement, more specifically defined self-actualization as "the desire to become more and more what one is, to become everything that one is capable of becoming."

Maslow recognized that the process of "becoming" has value apart from the end goal. In becoming, a person realizes what is valuable. It is these internal values that determine subsequent human choices and behavior, including self-recrimination.

These choices affect how you react to your situation. Have you lapsed into excessive focus on what others expect of you, or have you sustained a healthy and reasonable self-focus? Have you been able to continue the small steps that usually help you stay on track or has something diverted your energy or attention? What is the nature of your relationships? What stressors are weakening your resolve? Have you unwittingly lapsed into comparing yourself to others? The point is to notice changes in health or your body in thoughtful, compassionate, and non-judgmental ways, to reassess your goals and priorities, and to shift toward a healthier lifestyle.

Healthy, moderate living is a shift in worldview. "Losing weight shouldn't be about eating less," states Alisa Anokhina in her must-watch TED Talk on dieting. "Rather, it should be about thinking differently." It's a shift in how individuals manage meaning. It moves from the inside out, beginning with what people really want (internal), not what the culture (conditioning from parents or whatever) tells them is true (external). The focus changes from being motivated externally to an ideal (e.g., "I am now 122 pounds!") toward the process itself (e.g., "Over the last two months, I've exercised on average three times a week!").

This process is not about only one thing, but it is about becoming healthier and more self-aware. Yes, you can be happy on the road to health, even without perfect numbers popping up on the bathroom scale. Yes, on the road to being a healthier version of you, there will be dips, potholes, and rockslides. However, it's the pursuit of the daily journey, not the obsessive, never-ending drive for perfection, which permits good health.

PLANNING FOR THE LAPSE

"You are an amazing person. Look at how great you look!" is a common accolade doled out when a person loses weight. Value judgments, however, such as these, are potentially harmful. Loaded in the message is the missive, "You didn't look great before." The risk of ignoring the value of an individual's effort and missing the rewards of the process also occurs. When value is only assigned to the end result, product, outcome, score, or conclusion, much of life is missed, since most of living is in the process and not the outcome.

Even for the most highly motivated individuals, change doesn't occur immediately or without herculean effort. Real, lasting change is riddled with relapse and frustration. In fact, individuals must expect it—and plan for it.

Lapses are not failures. They are normal variants in human behavior. Setbacks are not proof of weakness, but only confirmation that you are normal and human. Missing an entire week of exercise is not failure. It happens.

Feeling frustrated by the confines of rigid dieting is the healthy you being expressed. Becoming bored with your diet or exercise regimen is ubiquitous. In fact, you should expect it and begin to plan for it. It is normal to want more freedom. Struggle in one area of health doesn't determine success or failure in other areas. Each day choices are available to you. The fundamental challenge is to identify what you want for your health and for yourself today and in each day?

In many ways, what this book is proposing is to permit normal human behavior. The 13-month-old, at first, has no interest in walking. Then, one day, he grabs the coffee table and pulls himself up for a few seconds. Then, he falls down. Maybe, he doesn't try it again for a week. Next thing you know, he's standing for a minute. The expectation is that he will topple over any moment. Finally, he does. Then, he gives up walking for crawling for a week. Next thing you know, he's walking. From that point forward, he begins to terrorize the house, given his newly acquired capacity to go where he wants to go.

With weight loss, there will be starts, stops, setbacks, and then progress. When you accept the way real people learn and grow, you can persist in your journey of becoming as healthy as you can be. Everyone will be challenged to tune out the lies of the culture, that generalized noise inside your head, comprised of an ensemble of voices, which declare "you will never look good enough." The more you cultivate the ability to live in the present, even after a day of setbacks, the more that the tyranny of thin will lose its chokehold on your happiness and, ultimately, your life.

Greater success can come from "living more in a more mindful place, a less confining place, and a place that allows greater expression of your unique character." It's not fixating on a number. By the same token, it is not saying "screw it," and giving up. To step into this middle space, in many ways, is to take a risk. In doing so, you might notice that what is most important to you may not be similarly valued by culture. Those people who are truly successful are able to set challenging goals for themselves that may run counter to popular cultural values, without sacrificing their own well-being or the well-being of others.

The measure of success may be more about what you overcome, than where you need to be. It is a belief that you can become a better you—always and that this objective is a goal worth pursuing. It is the belief that great progress can be achieved in relatively small steps, and that it is okay to change your mind about which steps are right for you.

A JOURNEY OF HOPE

Each person's path to health is unique. As such, small changes made today make for a better tomorrow. Considering a more middle range of options for living, indeed, transforms people, as the following two stories depict:

❑ *Story #1.* For the past three years, Jessica (the ballerina with the eating disorder) hasn't stepped on the weight-loss roller coaster. She has maintained a stable weight. In turn, her situation has led to stable physical, as well as mental, health. No longer is she bingeing or always preoccupied with her weight. She rarely lapses into the "Because I'm so fat and horrible, I'm not going to eat all week" mentality. Her blood pressure has dropped into a normal range. She doesn't engage in extreme workouts, but exercises five times a week, doing something she enjoys, dancing. She has found happier options that permit her to live more in the process of living.

❑ *Story #2.* A friend has a son who in his early teens and is arguably 30 pounds overweight. He is an athlete. At one time, he was one of the heaviest kids in his elementary school. A couple of years ago, though, he began putting on weight. He is above-average height for his age. At 13, the boy plays offensive line for an area football team and wrestles for his middle school. Even so, he has been ridiculed for his weight, even to the point of being bullied. His father once intervened by calling the vice-principal of the school to stop the humiliation dealt out by one particular boy to his son during lunch.

The past few years, his parents encouraged him to engage in healthy eating, but worked hard to respect him and his size, as it was. They tried to help him make healthier choices, when eating out or for his after-school snacks. They also avoided focusing on his weight and his diet-related numbers. Middle school is hard enough without the social burden of weight-related judgment, teasing, and bullying. Comments from his parents could only make things worse.

Recently, on a trip to Starbucks, his father asked him what he wanted. Normally, the boy asked for a peppermint hot chocolate. This time, he replied that he wanted a smoothie and actually said that he was trying to eat in a healthier way. His father was taken aback. Not long after, his son ordered water with lunch, a significant change from his previous usual order of a glass of lemonade or a bottle of Dr. Pepper.

He is still the biggest kid in his school. On the other hand, he is their kid, loved and respected by his parents at any weight. He remains physically active and increasingly aware of some available healthy eating options. Furthermore, he is able to make those decisions without being instructed to do so by parents. Hopefully, his healthier choices are motivated by an interest in health and improving self-awareness.

The BMI chart would still affirm his imperfection, since his BMI does not fall "within his ideal BMI percentile." More importantly, he is not on a diet. Furthermore, he is not oblivious to his weight or ignoring it. He is in a more middle place for himself, one that feels more right and more balanced for him—a scenario that is both helpful and hopeful.

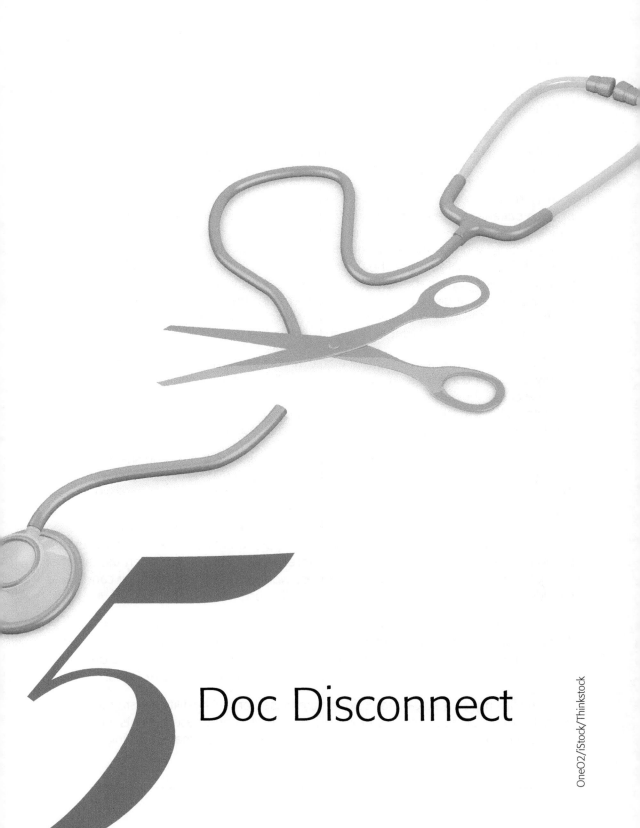

5

Doc Disconnect

On the way home from a basketball game one night, Trevor asked his mom if he could skip breakfast. He was eight years old. "I don't want to be as big as I am," he said. "I want to lose some pounds."

"Why do you want to lose weight?" his mom replied. It took a few more questions, but finally Trevor said, "The doctor called me *big* and *heavy*."

His annual physical exam was conducted the day before. Trevor said he felt bad after the appointment. He recalled the doctor saying, "For as big as you are, you really don't have a big stomach at all. You must just be stocky all over."

His mother was heartbroken. While physicians typically have the best interest of their patients at heart, the values of the culture can affect how doctors care for their patients. It's no wonder that patients dread being weighed at the beginning of appointments and fear the weight-related conversations that are sure to follow. Trevor is at risk for internalizing that he is somehow "fat," bad, or not normal. Internalized weight stigma increases the risk of more severe obesity, plummeting confidence, and the onset of eating disorders. Patients may feel that healthcare providers are quick to assume that they alone are personally responsible for their weight status and to advise them how to treat or correct their "weight" problem.

Granted, it is well documented that a modest weight reduction can improve a variety of health conditions, including blood pressure, serum cholesterol, and diabetic risk. Research, however, verifies the fact that some doctors stereotype overweight patients, although often unknowingly, as readily as does the culture. Sadly, it seems that the "thin fix" has made its way into the examination room.

Studies suggest that deriding individuals about their weight, size, and shape is the last socially acceptable form of prejudice. Is it at all surprising that healthcare providers share the same negative views of overweight individuals? One landmark study on obesity found that primary-care doctors are prone to characterize their obese patients as "awkward," "unattractive," "ugly," and "noncompliant." More than one-third of the physicians surveyed regarded obese individuals as "weak-willed," "sloppy," and "lazy." Medical students may be no less prejudiced. In a number of instances, obese patients are often the target of their jokes, believing that such patients are less worthy of care, because their condition is considered self-imposed and, in some cases, self-abuse.

The popular TV medical-drama *Grey's Anatomy* captured this bias in one episode. When a 700-pound man is admitted on a stretcher, Dr. Alex (a character in the show) pegs the patient as the villain and makes a joke at his expense: "I got a good one. What did they call the guy who was so fat, he couldn't get out of the house? Dead."

In reality, not all medical professionals are biased or feel hostility toward their obese patients. Many caring physicians treat their overweight and obese patients with dignity and respect, while helping them improve their health. Unfortunately, so ingrained are the weight-related biases in society that physicians and other healthcare providers may not be aware of some biases and their detrimental effects.

Research documents the prevalence of weight bias among doctors and its effects on patients. One study, for example, showed that physicians spend fewer minutes educating overweight patients, than they do with lower-weight patients, about health matters. Compared to appointments with thinner patients, physicians spend less time with obese patients, have less discussion with them, and admit that they don't intervene as much as they think they should.

Some physicians are less interested in treating obese patients, have more negative feelings about obese patients, doubt that obese patients will follow medical advice, and spend fewer minutes in consultation with them compared to their non-obese patients. Other research showed the existence of a higher BMI, associated with lower physician respect. In addition, it appears that physicians schedule fewer screenings for illnesses, such as cancer with patients who are overweight than with patients of average or low weight.

Is it surprising, then, when patients who are overweight or obese are less likely to return for recommended follow-up visits and additional evaluation, compared to non-obese patients? A more recent study found that doctors have less respect for their obese patients than they do for patients of normal weight. Furthermore, many physicians believe that "normal" patients are fixable, but not obese patients. Of the physicians surveyed, only 14 percent thought that they could actually help patients who are obese lose weight. Furthermore, less than half of them felt confident that their patients would be able to lose weight.

The lead researcher in another study, Mary Margaret Huizinga, M.D., M.P.H., also noticed this trend at work in a weight-loss clinic. In an interview, she recalls that patients "by the end of the visit would be in tears, saying no other physician talked with me like this before. No one listened to me. Many patients felt like because they were overweight, they weren't receiving the type of care other patients received."

It would be logical to hope that medical professionals who are specializing in obesity might be more sympathetic. Surprisingly, they're not. At a national conference on obesity, healthcare professionals were asked to assess their biases toward obese patients using the Implicit Association Test (IAT). This test is designed to detect the strength of a person's automatic associations between a particular concept and a specific attribute.

In this instance, the test asked participants to rate their beliefs about "fat" and "thin" people as either bad or good. The study, which focused on participants' personal, as well as professional, experiences with obesity, found that healthcare professionals implicitly were more prone to view obese patients as lazy, stupid, and worthless. The obvious question that arises from the findings of this investigation is if medical care providers cannot hurdle their biases and resist shaming patients, whom can patients trust with their health?

A simple Google search captures the outrage that people feel toward the medical community. One message board lit up with stories after a popular blogger, XO Jane, wrote a post indicting the medical community: "Dear Doctors, Quit with the Weight Bullying." The following are a few of the reader responses to her post:

- *My gynecologist told me that I'm getting too fat, and, perhaps, I should join the YMCA. I nodded in agreement, but, really he was the last person I wanted to hear tell me that I was fat and that I should do something about it. I was getting divorced, graduating from grad school, moving to an apartment, and suffering from a bit of postpartum depression. Instead of telling him off, I went home and ordered a pizza.*

- *I went to the doc because of painful TMJ keeping me awake for days—I was exhausted and in pain, and, for the first time, had a slightly above-norm blood pressure. She does not want to talk about my jaw. She, instead, tells me that I need to stop eating fast food (which—#1) She did not ask me if I eat and #2) I don't eat fast food more than a few times a year) and that I clearly need blood pressure meds. I try to explain my eating habits, that my blood pressure reading is unusual for me, and that the problem is my jaw pain. Her response was if I lost some weight and stopped eating so much fast food, I wouldn't be having this problem.*

- *I've had a lifetime of doctors telling me I'm too fat. Oh, except that one time when I was severely exercise anorexic (ran three miles a day and danced for four to eight hours a day) and ate nothing but lettuce and brown rice for six months. When I was weighed in at the doctor's office, they praised me for my weight loss and how "good" I was doing, without asking for any details on my "eating" or exercising habits.*

Most people have heard countless similar stories. Medical-care providers may blame a patient's weight, rather than a nasty fall, for a patient's sprained ankle or blown knee. In turn, they may dismiss more aggressive care, make inaccurate assumptions, or wrongly assign blame.

I once counseled a patient who was a cancer survivor. One year after surgery and completing chemotherapy, she was on the road to recovery. Her labs were good; she was in the clear. At the time, her weight was 65 pounds less than her highest adult weight, but she was still (according to a height-weight chart) 60 pounds overweight. During a consult with her internist, he remarked on her good lab results. A moment later he added, "You don't deserve this." His point to her was that someone who is overweight doesn't deserve good news or good health.

Despite numerous studies showing that overweight conditions and good health can co-exist, that obesity does not necessarily shorten a person's life, and that dieting does not guarantee happiness, this blaming and shaming continues to reverberate with too many individuals: "You don't deserve anything good because you're not good. You're fat."

It is also what prompts many patients to "walk out of the office, and never go back." For individuals of any size, no matter what they do to improve their overall health, the scales, height-weight charts, and BMI data rule the day. As such, many patients say it feels like whatever they do is never enough.

Recently, a patient, Michael, described his distress concerning a marital therapy appointment that he had attended with his wife the previous day. He and his wife had been seeing this therapist for some time to work on improving their communication in the relationship and addressing Michael's frustrations around being the "sole bread winner" throughout the history of their relationship.

Michael, who had recently gained weight, was admonished by his wife and their marriage therapist for his eating patterns. They declared his eating to be out of control and suggested that he eat less. Michael was hard working, brilliant, and highly accomplished in his chosen profession, but his health had been poor for some time. He battled life-long depression, addictions, asthma, untreatable immune-related illnesses, and chronic pain. In an effort to take care of himself, he had multiple care providers, frequent doctor's appointments, used a variety of medications daily, underwent periodic tests and procedures, and worked to maintain recovery from addictions.

Michael had lapsed to smoking over the past six months, but had stopped again three weeks prior to this particular appointment with his marital therapist under the advice of his doctor. Michael admitted his eating had been poorly controlled, especially during the weeks in which he was suffering intense nicotine withdrawal. His wife and therapist "intended" to help him eat well and lose weight. Unfortunately, he left that appointment feeling reprimanded and reminded that he was "not good enough." His motivation for self-care and healthy eating plummeted.

A physician's training readies them to discuss the numbers associated with the risks of obesity: high blood pressure, high blood sugar, and high cholesterol. On the other hand, given the limited amount of training in the psychosocial components of obesity, physicians may not know how to engage patients in a more helpful manner about weight-related health. As a result, the physician defaults to "weight-loss talk."

Certainly, the vast majority of physicians are smart, good, caring people. The situation involving patients who need to lose weight, however, appears in some cases to confound them, as reflected in their comments about the issue. "Other than listing the risks and reminding them what they are doing to themselves, what can I do about it?" "The patient is not motivated to lose weight." "They just aren't trying." In reality, it is often easier for physicians to focus on the numbers and the reminders. Such a tactic may be more consistent with the traditional medical model that entails identifying what is broken and prescribing a fix.

Assumptions regarding overeating and insufficient physical activity can dominate the thinking in the physician's office, despite the unique individual differences that exist between patients. The reality is that some individuals gain or lose weight more easily than others, based on their genetic background. Unfortunately, there is not one program or one remedy that is appropriate for all patients or clients.

Even if patients hypothetically aren't doing anything right, doctors can provide good information, discuss the patient's interests and needs, and offer encouragement and support. If nothing else, their patients did successfully find their way to the office and could be encouraged to return.

The physician could, for example, ask how their patient feels about their weight, body, shape, and health. They could also inquire about their patient's self-care and ask if the patient is interested in additional information or support. Physicians can acknowledge their patient's efforts while validating the difficulty and complexity of the weight-loss process. Furthermore, they can highlight the patient's progress and accomplishments—even those the patient might not recognize.

Physicians are in an optimal position to participate in their patient's healthcare, align themselves with the goals of their patients, and, in the process, become part of the solution. Healthcare providers can empower their patients to make well-informed and healthier choices, and even more importantly, not to throw in the proverbial towel.

It is a fact that blaming and shaming intended to motivate, can create a downward, negative spiral of thoughts, emotions, and behavior, which may end in avoidance of healthcare. The following is an example of an avoidance cycle in this situation:

- Doctors recommend weight loss to improve health.
- The patients make a return visit to their physician, during which they are weighed. According to the scale, their weight has not changed upward or downward since their previous doctor's visit.
- The doctors repeat the message about the importance of weight reduction.
- The patients feel criticized and ashamed and that their efforts to improve their nutrition and exercise are insufficiently acknowledged.
- The doctors tell the patients that they hope to see more improvement.
- Outwardly, the patients agree, but, inwardly, they feel reprimanded.
- The doctors document each patient's weight and the fact that the weight consultation was completed.
- The patients return home, feeling a bit defeated. The patients vow to curb their diet and get more exercise. On the other hand, the patients become increasingly preoccupied with food. The patients already dread the next visit and weigh-in.
- The patients try to rally and make changes, but their efforts do not result in the prescribed weight loss. The patients disappoint themselves, as well as worry they will disappoint the doctor.
- The patients, having tried to lose weight on several previous occasions, feel overwhelmed about the lengthy and challenging nature of the weight-loss journey and search for motivation to diet—again.

- Realizing that weight loss may take some time and not wanting to disappoint the physician yet again or be reminded of their failings, the patients either reschedule their appointment date or cancel the appointment until further notice.
- Later, the doctor's office calls to encourage a return visit. Feeling embarrassed, the patients do not return the call. Avoidance feels better in the moment than facing the anxiety associated with the appointment and the enormity of the effort necessary to attend doctor's appointments and work toward weight loss.
- Medical conditions left untreated may become more complex and damaging. If the next office visit is driven out of medical need, the doctor may be frustrated with the patient's delay in getting into the office for the recommended re-evaluation.
- The patients sense the doctor's frustration and become reluctant to return to the office again, unless it is absolutely necessary.
- The doctors want to help their patients, but are aware of the fact that their effectiveness is limited if they cannot see the patients in the office.
- The doctors may feel unmotivated to spend a large amount of time and energy to consult with a patient who may be unlikely to return for regular visits or who may appear to be "unmotivated to change."
- The patients may feel dismissed, further challenging the patient-physician connection, which reduces their level of motivation to return to the doctor's office.

In this moment, it's not just about "calories in, calories out." It's not just about willpower. It's not just merely a lack of self-control or insufficient nutritional information. In this moment, it's, at least, one part systemic. The very system upon which patients depend for their healthcare reinforces their deepest fears: that they can't change, that their efforts toward self-care are insufficient, that their physician doesn't really hear or care for them, and that they may not be worthy of being healthy.

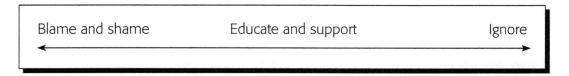

| Blame and shame | Educate and support | Ignore |

WEIGHTISM AND ITS CONSEQUENCES

A pediatrician told her son that the red mark under his arm was only something that happens to "fat people." Discrimination is, according to the dictionary, "the practice of unfairly treating a person or group of people differently from other people." One recently conducted study concluded that weight discrimination may increase the risk for obesity, rather than motivating individuals to lose weight.

Another study found that eating is a common coping response in the face of stress, with 79 percent of 2,449 women admitting they increased the amount of food that they ate to cope with the stigma of being overweight. Assessed in 2006 and again in 2010, participants in this investigation who experienced weight discrimination were more than twice as likely to become obese by the follow-up assessment. Obese participants who were on the receiving end of perceived weight discrimination in 2006 were "not" motivated to lose weight. Instead, they were more likely to remain obese at the 2010 visit than those individuals who did not experience discrimination.

Discrimination can have a number of negative consequences. Not only can it add an additional layer of burden to daily living, it can lower the individual's level of self-confidence. Furthermore, in some cases, it can leave people wanting to give up or avoid subsequent healthcare.

"Doctor shopping," which can disrupt continuity and quality of healthcare, is another outcome of the protective avoidance cycle. According to Yale's Rudd Center's director of research and weight stigma initiatives, Dr. Rebecca Puhl, 19 percent of adults and 24 percent of parents of obese children would avoid future medical appointments, if they perceived a doctor had used stigmatized language to describe their weight or their child's weight. Furthermore, 21 percent of adults and 35 percent of parents would switch doctors if this situation happened to them.

Another study that examined 21,000 Blue Cross Blue Shield claims found that overweight patients were 23 percent more likely to have had visits with five or more primary care doctors within a two-year period. Obese patients, meanwhile, had a 52 percent greater chance of having been seen by an unduly large number of doctors, who compared with normal-weight patients. "Such research does not prove that obese patients are getting worse care because of physician bias," states lead author of the study, Kimberly A. Gudzune, MD, MPH, "but it does suggest that many of these patients are experiencing unsatisfactory relationships with their doctors." Overweight and obese patients who shopped around for doctor were also 85 percent more likely to end up in the emergency room for healthcare than the non-overweight and non-obese individual.

An adult female, a 40-year-old patient who was employed full-time, was close to family and friends, and worked, doing what she loved. She had struggled with obesity and related health complications for over two decades and had elected to undergo bariatric surgery. She was referred to a behavioral health clinic for a physician-required, pre-surgical psychological evaluation. Once her evaluation was finished, she was found to be psychologically able to make decisions about surgery and her healthcare.

Her surgery was completed several weeks later, just prior to a holiday weekend. A family member had found our business card in her coat pocket and gave us a call. She had been discharged from the hospital, but called two days later, complaining of abdominal pain. The doctor's office told her the pain was common and likely due to gas.

On Sunday, with the patient still in pain, her relative took her to the ER. She was examined and then discharged. She was told to follow up with her physician after the holiday weekend. On Sunday evening, she was transported to the hospital, via ambulance, where she underwent extensive emergency surgery and died early Monday morning.

Some patients who are obese might be turned away before beginning a relationship with a physician. A provocative CBS news report, "Fat-Phobic Doctors Refuse to Treat Obese Patients: Is That Fair?" cites the rise of a "no-fatties-allowed" policy by physicians. While the reasons vary for implementation of the policy—for example, either the examination equipment isn't large enough or the obese patients are a liability—the policy seems to be another form of flagrant weight discrimination.

Ida Davidson, self-admittedly a "little overweight," captured the nation's attention when she publicly took to task Dr. Helen M. Carter for implementing a screening policy that rejects patients who top 200 pounds. During her second visit to Dr. Carter, Davidson was informed of the new policy. "She didn't care about my health that day. I think she just cared that I was a liability to her maybe and too much work for her," Davidson told Boston news radio station WCVB.

A blogger who covered Ms. Davidson's story on *Jezebel*, a blog aimed at women's interests, poses, "In medical school, the motto is primum non nocere—first, do no harm. Isn't there psychological and emotional harm done when a doctor—someone you're attempting to have an intimate, deeply personal relationship with—refuses to examine you because your body isn't thin enough? What if a patient is turned away and is so humiliated … she avoids seeking medical attention?"

The shame-game never produces winners. On the other hand, even the best and brightest in the medical community still "give it a go." Ethicist Daniel Callahan, president emeritus of the health ethics think tank The Hastings Center, is rallying for a type of "stigmatization-lite." He believes that shaming the obese will prompt weight loss. "It is hard to imagine that much progress can occur toward solutions for obesity," he writes, "unless we bring some form of social pressure to bear against it."

Really, "some form of social pressure?" While Callahan recognizes that such an approach can be a difficult line to walk (i.e., such stigmatization could turn into overt discrimination), he still wants to give it a try. He urges healthcare professionals to awaken obese individuals to their condition with a variety of questions, including the following:

- If you are overweight or obese, are you *pleased* with the way you look?
- Are you *happy* that your added weight has made many ordinary activities, such as walking up a long flight of stairs, more difficult?
- Fair or not, do you know that many people look down upon those excessively overweight or obese, often, in fact, discriminating against them and making fun of them or calling them *lazy* and *lacking in self-control?*

The social pressure that Callahan calls for is bullying. His array of assumptions are patently false.

Assumption #1: "You will be pleased with your appearance if you are thin." Wrong.

Assumption #2: "Suffering and discontent motivates behavioral health compliance." Wrong.

Assumption #3: "Changing your weight or appearance will ensure that you will not be discriminated against." Wrong.

Assumption #4: "You, the patient, might not notice that I am discriminating against you by speaking to you this way, and you might believe that I really can help you take good care of your health." Wrong.

In reality, the social pressures that include shame, blame, threats, and false promises have already patronized a number of physician offices, homes, and schools across the nation for some time. Even the most optimistic person could conclude that this approach is not working as intended.

If "social pressures" were the fix, this country would have crashing rates of obesity. It doesn't. The weight and diet reminders are everywhere. Standing between their heavier self and their idealized self, many obese individuals endlessly ruminate over each lapse or failure.

One client, who is struggling with escalating weight, recently returned from a trip to Italy. When asked her how the trip was, she replied, "Horrible! I ate too much pasta!" I heard myself asking why she would not want to eat pasta in Italy?

Another patient not too long ago announced on a Monday morning that the weekend was a failure, because she "ate Cheetos." I asked him if he aspired to a life without "Cheetos." In fact, food and eating are wonderful ways to celebrate custom and tradition. Why would anyone want to live their life without joy and pleasure? As a rule, animals and humans usually do not prefer to sustain behaviors that are depriving and punishing.

The current culture's diet-related expectations seem enormous. The guilt is not only piled high, it is unnecessary. It is not commonly understood that room exists for variation in diet, level of activity, and related behaviors on the journey to improved health. Medical professionals who intentionally or unintentionally shame their obese patients only add to the cauldron of self-hatred.

Some weight specialists, however, are firing back, calling for physicians to become allies of their patients. The Patient Promise, developed by medical students at John Hopkins, is one such initiative. Medical providers who sign the pact commit to support their patients who are struggling with obesity, to identify and guard themselves from weight prejudices, and to respect their patients, regardless of their body size.

It may be helpful to remember that at least half, and likely more than half, of the patients that a physician treats will be overweight or obese. Furthermore, many patients might fear becoming so.

UNLOCKING THE MYSTERY

I was recently invited to lecture to medical school residents at a large university on eating disorders. They were weeks away from graduation and were already planning their celebrations. I had arrived early for my lecture and chose to sit in on the preceding lecture, which was on obesity. Two and one half hours in length, the presentation summarized the guidelines for the top 10 most popular diets in the United States today. Subsequently, I asked about course work or other lectures on obesity and was informed that this lecture was the only class dedicated to this topic.

Biases aside, some physicians have little formal training in the social and emotional complexity of the various weight conditions, eating behavior, and obesity. Historically, it has not been customary for physicians to study the principles of socio-cultural and psychological factors associated with behavioral change. It's not that physicians don't have the desire to help individuals of all sizes with supporting good health. Doing so, however, in the current culture is an art that many physicians have not yet perfected.

When the Strategies to Overcome and Prevent (STOP) Obesity Alliance surveyed 290 primary-care physicians, it found that 89 percent of the respondents want to help their patients lose weight. Equally enlightening, most physicians recognize that it's their responsibility to do so. On the other hand, they often don't know what to say to these patients. Their training in dealing with weight-related conditions is sparse, if not non-existent. Seventy-two percent of physicians noted that no one in their practice had been trained to deal with such issues.

When patients have questions about weight, they, initially, often turn to their physician, who is, typically, a good choice for the first conversation. Patients want to know both what to do and how to do it. The question arises, however, whether re physicians are able to provide the help that patients seek. According to a Harris poll of 1002 patients, only one-third of those individuals who were told to lose weight reported that their physicians discussed how they should lose the weight.

Surprisingly, the one place patients expect to find answers is surprisingly little help. Christine Ferguson, director of the STOP Alliance, says, "It's like going to the doctor and being told, 'Oh, your blood sugar is high,' and that's the end of the conversation." Furthermore, she goes on to state, "Doctors don't feel they have good information to give. They feel that they don't have adequate tools to address this problem."

Until recently, when the American Medical Association (AMA) made the landmark decision to officially recognize obesity as a disease, physicians were more reluctant to spend time discussing obesity as a stand-alone issue. According to Dr. Richard H. Carmona, former U.S. Surgeon General and STOP chairman, "Even if they had those precious extra minutes, many would still be missing the needed information about weight-loss tools and existing programs."

Physicians could use more tools and options for managing weight, such as binge-eating support groups, nutrition education support, meal planning, specialized psychotherapy, exercise specialists, no-cost or low-cost walking groups, medication support for appetite control (e.g., Vyvanse, Abbott Pharmaceuticals, FDA approved, February 2015), mood management, parent-child feeding practice education and support, etc.

Effective programs and support are difficult to find, slow-going, difficult to develop, hard to motivate patients to engage, and time-consuming to monitor. Dealing with the complexity of obesity takes time, resources, and specialty training, which physicians often fine in short supply.

Hopefully, with the passage of the AMA's resolution on obesity, insurers will increasingly fund consultations exclusively related to weight. The underlying objective of the measure is to reimburse a physician for the time they spend treating obesity as a complex problem. Specifically, the AMA resolved "that providers receive appropriate financial support and payment from third-party payers, thus ensuring that providers have an incentive to manage the complex diseases associated with obesity."

Morgan Downey, an advocate for people with obesity and publisher of the online *Downey Obesity Report* reiterates, "I think you will probably see … physicians taking obesity more seriously, counseling their patients about it." Unfortunately, the promise of more available reimbursement comes at a time when the medical community is experiencing a reduction in the minutes and dollars allocated for services overall, larger patient co-pay, larger deductibles, and, for the physician, higher costs for medical education and medical practice than ever in history.

If physicians are to be able to straddle the duo roles of both counselor and physician, proper training is imperative. In ever-increasing numbers, medical programs are requiring that their students participate in mandatory obesity education courses. In that regard, the medical school of Wake Forest University is leading the charge. After taking a hard look at medical training across the country, the school determined that of the academic medical centers (including Wake Forest Baptist—an academic medical center that is affiliated with Wake Forest University), only a small number of institutions "are providing adequate, effective training" to their students in assisting obese patients.

While obesity prevention is a staple of medical training, public health sciences professor at Wake Forest Baptist, Dr. Mara Vitolins, concluded most coursework doesn't help students identify their biases toward or develop their skills in treating overweight and obese patients. According to Dr. Vitolins, obesity and related bias should be added as a rotation for all physicians in training.

Wake Forest's training transcends several years of coursework. It encourages students to face their stereotypes through use of the Weight Implicit Association Test. It also helps to develop an elementary empathy for overweight individuals in students through viewing a documentary that discusses the challenges that obese individuals face in daily living, in interacting with the health system, and with their yo-yoing weight over time.

Baylor College of Medicine in Houston is another school that is incorporating exposure to weight bias in medicine throughout its four-year curriculum. In addition, thousands of health professionals have tapped into the free online, continuing medical education course offered by the Yale University Rudd Center for Food Policy and Obesity. Yale's course is designed to help healthcare providers dispense better care for their overweight patients.

COMPLEXITY IN A SIMPLE-FIX CULTURE

With regard to training physicians on how to effectively and appropriately deal with weight matters, some progress has been made. In fact, a few medical schools currently include obesity training in their curriculum. As such, medical professionals are inching toward recognizing the fact that weight conditions do not exist separately from the individual; nor do they exist separately from our culture.

Those physicians without training, however, are more likely to be swayed by ingrained stereotypes. Lock-step with culture, these physicians tend to view the problem as one-dimensional. Fat is the problem, and no fat is the solution. Such a simplistic mindset leads to the common cure for the average overweight person: increase the amount that you exercise and decrease how much you eat. On occasion, surgery is the prescribed lifeboat recommended for survival: "You need bariatric surgery." All too rarely do these doctors ask their patients about their eating patterns, their expectations, their dieting history, their psychological well-being, how they view exercise, how difficult it will be for them to incorporate exercise into their daily regimen, or what medical conditions might make exercise difficult, if not impossible, for them to sustain.

Instead, physicians should consider the needs of their patients three-dimensionally: understanding where they come from, where they are currently, and where they want to go. With that understanding, the patients know what they can solve easily, what's going to take more work, and what resources they may need to make the desired changes. This approach is what every patient deserves, but not every patient receives.

With regard to bariatric surgery, extracting the fat and fat cells through such a medical treatment may be productive and less time-consuming than engaging in other options. In fact, several surgical interventions, such as gastric bypass, bands, and sleeves, have had dramatic and immediate effects on normalizing blood sugar and correcting diabetic conditions. On the other hand, surgery has its own risks, including infection, surgical complication, excessive malabsorption, anemia, vitamin deficiency, and possible death.

Once they undergo the procedure, some individuals may need additional surgical modification. Some individuals may be at a greater risk for alcohol-related or other addictions. After their surgery, other individuals may be presented with unwanted mood- or anxiety-related issues. Furthermore, excessive gas, bloating, indigestion, nausea, and gastrointestinal distress are all common, but often treatable, post-surgery symptoms. All factors considered, patients enjoy the weight change and the better appetite control that occurs after bariatric surgery. More recent surgical procedures, especially those with a permanent by-pass effect, appear to result in more permanent weight loss.

As a new and inexperienced psychologist working with clients who had frustrations with their weight, I understood how hard and courageously they strove to battle their bodies' inclination to gain weight quickly and easily, as well as to then hold onto it forever. In all honesty, however, I was guilty of having an insufficient level of appreciation for the unique challenges with which each client struggles. I incorrectly assumed that several weight-related factors, such as interest in eating, ability to feel full, preoccupation with food, and degree of hunger, varied little from person to person.

I continued to hold that attitude until I was pregnant with my first child. One day, as my husband and I embarked on our half-hour commute, I was overcome with intense hunger. I asked my husband to turn off at the next exit, so I could get something to eat. He passed the exit. I asked again, this time with growing panic. He passed another exit. At that point, we were only 20 minutes from home. Surely, he assumed, I could wait until we reached home.

With each passing request and as each exist passed, I felt more painfully hungry, which only fueled my anger. "If you don't stop at the next exit, I'm going to punch you!" I exclaimed. Furthermore, I meant it.

I understood in that moment that all hunger was not created equal. I learned in a small way that biochemical and physiological mechanisms can powerfully drive the obese condition. I also gained an awareness that these mechanisms may be powerful entities unto themselves, with minds all their own. I had failed to appreciate the fact that the intensity of the signals and the drive to eat may have extreme variation in each person. I gained an appreciation for the need to refrain from assuming that I "understand" something, before I take more time to learn.

Not every doctor will become an expert on obesity and related issues, such as hormone production, energy metabolism, and appetite. On the other hand, most physicians must be able to appreciate the biology and chemistry of various weight conditions. Furthermore, they must be able to advise their patients about what they might expect and be frustrated by with their efforts to lose weight or why, for example, they might be hungry during a period of weight loss. It's not because they are crazy or weak-willed, but because their body is starving. In fact, it's doing what it is supposed to do—kicking up the appetite as a signal to eat more, thereby providing protection until the body's metabolism restabilizes.

In fact, physicians should be trained to respond constructively to patient questions about exercise, nutrition, and weight and to assist their patients in becoming more knowledgeable. Furthermore, healthcare providers should receive training in specialized communication techniques that are designed to help patients feel informed, but not shamed or reprimanded about their weight-related concerns.

As such, the improvements in the way that members of the healthcare community communicate with their obese patients may need to occur in terms of "how" that information is best delivered, as well as in terms that reflect the physician's ability to withstand making assumptions or reaching premature judgments. To a degree, motivating better self-care in an individual will depend on preserving the patient's self-confidence and acknowledging the patient's efforts and small successes.

What about exercise for weight loss? In 2009, The American College of Sports Medicine published a position stand on this topic. It was concluded that while many obese people may have to start at a relatively low-intensity level while exercising, they should try to exercise longer and more often in order to reach a greater total expenditure of energy.

Because energy is used to transport a person's body weight, people who walk use a similar amount of energy to walk the same distance. Even if they walk faster or slower, the energy per mile walked is similar. In other words, although individuals use more energy per minute when they walk faster, they walk fewer minutes to cover the same distance.

Furthermore, the distance walked per day or week can be accumulated over several walks. An individual doesn't have to undertake all of the exercise in a single session. As a result, the overweight/obese person should be encouraged to walk as far as possible each day to increase the total amount of energy expended. Once their tolerance for the demands being placed on their body by the exercise improves, they can walk faster to cover the same distance in less time or walk a greater distance in the same time.

Healthcare professionals may not realize that the five-days-a-week of physical activity recommended by the Centers for Disease Control and Prevention and The American College of Sports Medicine is substantially more than what most adults in the United States currently are able to accomplish. When obese individuals finally decide to take up exercising, often what the doctor prescribes is too much, too difficult, and too long.

For example, I once had a client who was so deconditioned that he exercised three times a day for very short periods, rather than the normative five times a week for a half hour at a time. His intensity and duration levels during these moments were much lower because his tolerance was much lower. The key point that should be noted, in this instance, is that by manipulating the frequency, intensity, duration, and mode, of the exercise bout, an individual can be helped to burn stored fat more efficiently.

The get-slim-and–fit-quick promises of infomercials, like P90X and Insanity Workout, are unsustainable for most people, given the risk of injury, the strain, and the level of exhaustion. In fact, such exercise routines are impossible to do safely for almost all obese individuals. Even relatively fit individuals experience burnout when the regimen is too difficult.

Everyone knows, from personal experience, that exercise that is not pleasant will less likely be repeated. For example, jogging three days a week, when all you can think about doing is stopping, is not likely to be sustained over time. In fact, individuals are more likely to look forward to working up a sweat if the activity is enjoyable or at least some specific component of the activity is particularly pleasant (e.g., visiting with friends, relishing the outdoor air, feeling a post-workout stress relief, time away for self-care, the fun of movement, or the challenge of competition).

The fact is that an individual doesn't need that much exercise to experience its benefits. On a scale ranging from point A (no activity) to point D (athletic activity), getting from point A to point B may require minimal effort, when compared to getting from point B to point D. The resultant health benefits, however, may not be that much more. The key factor to remember is that people don't have to be competitive athletes to get the health benefits of exercise.

Too often, however, doctors fail to acknowledge that "victory" for an obese person may mean getting from point A to point B, especially if that individual hasn't reached their BMI target. Similarly, a number of physicians may not fully appreciate the fact that 70 to 85 percent of a person's daily caloric expenditure is not a function of how much that individual exercises. In reality, it is a function of the demands of daily living. These demands have steadily fallen since the early 1900s—especially since 1971. In that regard, the industrial revolution (which led to reliance on machinery, instead of manual labor), automated transportation, and even an increased use of technology (e.g., computers, remote controls, cell phones, and telecommuting, etc.) have all contributed to a reduction in how much energy individuals expend daily.

While the level of daily energy expenditure continues to fall, calorie-dense, inexpensive, readily-available, pre-cooked, and bite-sized foods (that individuals don't even have to balance on a fork or cut with a knife!) are increasingly available. As such, these two factors collectively create a perfect environment for weight gain and present huge challenges for weight stability or weight loss.

PRESCRIBING HOPE

Recently, I attended a conference sponsored by Health at Every Size (HAES), an organization that promotes self-acceptance at any shape, weight, or size. During a breakout session, I was seated at a table with six other attendees, a group that reflected varying shapes and sizes. Our assignment was to "discuss an uncomfortable physician- or medical-related experience that was weight-related."

The group was well-educated and well-intended in weight-related matters. Before one particular individual shared her story, however, she looked at me and said, "Well you won't understand my experience because you have never had a weight problem, so there is no point in my telling my story. You won't get it."

In the most diplomatic manner I could muster at the time, I said, "I am here. I am attending the conference because I want to learn. I want to be as well-informed as possible. It is probably true that I cannot completely know or fully appreciate all that you might have experienced or all that you might describe in your story. But, I am here because I want to understand and want to be a constructive part of making things better. I want to listen." She quietly reflected for a moment and then shared her story.

While anecdotes and statistics paint a relatively bleak picture of the relationship between overweight patients and their physicians, I believe it can look different. It is important to note that physicians do not have to manage these issues perfectly. Truthfully, they will improve the likelihood that they can have a positive influence on the situation if they position themselves appropriately, by simply "aligning" their efforts with those of their patients.

It will be beneficial for physicians to take a moment, whenever possible, to hear more about the perspectives or preferences of their patients. Physicians can learn a lot by listening to them. In fact, it can be invaluable for physicians to learn more about the goals of their patients, as well as what might be interfering with them making better progress.

For many medical professionals, the solution to obesity is obvious—eat less and exercise more. Frustration settles in when the perceived next step is too difficult and overwhelming for the patient to take.

An episode of the television show *The Dog Whisperer* reminded me that force and reproach work against progress. The dog trainer, Cesar Millan, was called in to help the owner of a police dog that had a phobia of walking on linoleum floors. When Cesar arrived, the police handler demonstrated the dog's ability to walk on carpet, hardwood floors, concrete, and tile. Jack, the dog, however, put on the brakes at the linoleum.

After several more demonstrations, Cesar accepted the challenge to correct this behavior. He then took Jack for a walk. When he and Jack got to the linoleum, Jack stood firmly planted at the doorway. Cesar tugged at the leash, and said, "Let's go." Still no movement. He gave another tug and released the tension on the leash. Finally, Cesar tugged once more, and Jack crossed the linoleum floor.

Later in the show, Cesar explained that incessant pulling on the leash conveys the message that "This situation must be really bad, otherwise, they wouldn't keep pulling me like this." Cesar further explained that tugging in the direction that the trainer wants the dog to move but then releasing the tension on the leash imparts "confidence" that the dog will be able to move in the desired direction.

Individuals of all sizes have received the "you need to do more," "you need to try harder," and "you are hurting yourself" messages too many times in their lives. The blame and criticism does not motivate better self-care. As a rule, doctors tend to be loved when their patients feel that they have been on the receiving end of the time, attention, and care provided by their physicians. All factors considered, most patients have no interest in where their family doctor went to medical school, whether their physician was top of the class, or whether their doctor has published an article in a referred medical journal. Instead, patients value how their physician spends time listening, calming fears, and answering seemingly trivial questions, as well as helping to collaboratively determine what the "next plan" for them will be.

In reality, it's time for an improved approach to doctor-patient relations. Hopefully, in this new mindset, medical professionals will champion patients, despite their weight; instill confidence in their ability to embrace essential life changes; and will impart an attitude of hope concerning a life of health. At that point, perhaps, patients will begin taking the somewhat frightening first steps toward a lifetime of health.

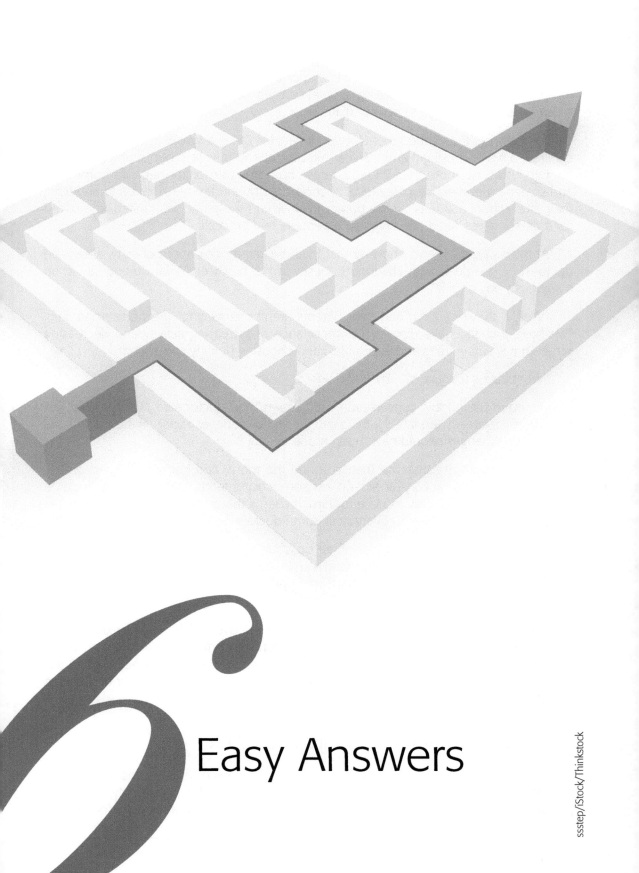

6 Easy Answers

Recently, a friend attended her son's end-of-the-season soccer party. As the boys romped around, she was drawn into a quiet conversation with the quintessential soccer mom, who also happens to be a pediatrician.

My friend is the embodiment of suburbia. Her car is a white Toyota Sienna. Her children, a 15-year-old girl and 13-year-old boy, attend private schools. She works just enough hours, no more than 25, so she can be home to monitor her kid's homework and screen time, watchdog their level of social activity, and taxi her children to and from their after-school activities. At the burger joint, where the party was hosted, she opted for a dressing-less salad piled high with peppers and broccoli.

At the party, my friend, knowing that I was writing a book about obesity, asked the doctor how she deals with childhood obesity in her practice: "What do you say to an overweight boy or girl?"

"Well, if they're young, and their parents aren't overweight," the pediatrician said, "we have a chance. We discuss the importance of increasing activity and decreasing screen time, eating fruits and vegetables, and choosing healthy snacks."

"What about teenagers?" my friend asked.

"If you're having this conversation with a teen," the doctor said, "then you've lost the battle. It's already too late. Nothing can be said or done, especially if the parents are overweight. Changes should have been made already."

My friend told me that she then scanned the room, and her eyes landed on the one overweight boy, a 13-year-old, on her son's soccer team. She said she wondered if the doctor thought it was too late for him. It seems that the cultural axiom "It's never too late," may have a weight covenant in some doctors' offices.

My friend said she also thought of her boss's teenage daughter, who is overweight. Over a decade, her parents had invested a small fortune in figuring out why the weight won't come off, including a trip to one of the premier medical institutions in the world. The teenager had attempted to lose weight over and over again.

Is it too late for her? Furthermore, what about the overweight latchkey kids whose parents work double shifts and can't make it home in time to fix a balanced meal, monitor their screen time, and encourage them to engage in physical activity. *Is it too late for them?* Is there hope for the 14-year-old, 47-year-old, or 76-year-old, whose climbing weight wasn't curbed by age 12?

WHEN ALL IS DARK, LOOK IN THE DARK

Hopelessness has been the story of obesity. With each failed "This is it!" diet, hopelessness seeps deeper into an individual's psyche. Not surprisingly, for many people, it can feel like the odds are stacked against them. Visit after visit, doctors see the results of the pursuit of thin and repetitive diet attempts—increased weight gain after weight loss, depression, diabetes, and heart disease, to name just a few. Hopelessness and despair can follow.

Hope is pilfered by peers, friends, and family members. They communicate, either overtly or inadvertently, that the overweight person is a disappointment, and they should just try harder. Their prevailing message is that: "If you'd just lose 30 more pounds." Her doctor echoes similar sentiments: "Maybe, if you exercised more, you could lose those 30 extra pounds," as if the 65 pounds she already dropped were nothing. Defeated, she weighs her options: the diet, which has betrayed her time and again, or the bowl of ice cream. *I will eat the ice cream, while I consider my options*," she thinks. *Why keep trying?* It's no wonder that overweight or obese people are at greater risk for depression, anxiety, low self-esteem, and poor body image.

Healthcare professionals are similarly beaten down by obesity's apparent endless cycling challenge. Weight bias exists among doctors and other healthcare professionals. Weight bias is ubiquitous, even among trusted professionals, like the family practice doctor. The promises of "thin," sold to us by American culture, exist in every corner of life.

In the previous chapters, the case was made that in the United States, people who are overweight are "falsely" associated with a lack of willpower, poor self-control, a lack of nutritional knowledge, and even with stupidity. Conversely, thin is more often associated with power, control, success, and intelligence. Even those professionals who are not biased and hold healthier perspectives on these matters may weary at the long slog toward health for those individuals who are overweight.

Even when change happens, the shift can be virtually imperceptible. Furthermore, in the American culture, looks are what matters to most. Like it is for everyone, it can be difficult for physicians and other healthcare providers to stay upbeat, when, statistically, approximately one out of three adult patients and one in five pediatric patients are obese, many of whom are confronted by the correlating health problems, like diabetes, heart disease, high blood pressure, sleep disorders, and joint problems. When patients return heavier year after year, it can feel futile for a physician to point out the government's "My Plate" recommendations and inquire about the patient's level of physical activity. Obligated to check the box that says they've discussed the patient's weight, many physicians ask the mandatory questions and offer the stock array of weight-loss recommendations. More often than not, many, like the pediatrician, believe it's too late.

Tragically, physicians who feel that a patient's obese condition is hopeless may verbally or silently convey that message through their actions—or lack thereof. To dig at the root of obesity and offer personalized support and resources is a time-consumer that many physicians *think* they can't afford and don't believe that will make a difference. To some physicians, counseling an obese patient may seem outside the scope of what's possible in a single, 15-minute visit. Others may wonder where actual medicine comes into play.

Medicine can be a powerful tool in treating obesity, when applied at key moments of the process. Prescribing a pill, a diet, or surgery without attending to the larger picture, however, may be shortsighted. A pill can't change genetic predisposition. A diet won't help someone with no support at home or a history of an eating disorder. Surgery doesn't solve the issue of lack of exercise. The doctor can diagnose and prescribe, but will the patient hear the advice, feel understood, know the advice is appropriate for their goals, and return a year later in a healthier state?

The story of "The Lost Ring," by the ancient Persian philosopher Mullah Nasreddin, illustrates how some physicians and healthcare providers may approach patients and their weight: *Mullah lost his ring in the living room. He searched for it for a while, but since he could not find it, he went out into the yard and began to look there. His wife, who saw what he was doing, asked, "Mullah, you lost your ring in the room. Why are you looking for it in the yard?" Mullah stroked his beard and said, "The room is too dark, and I can't see very well. I came out to the courtyard to look for my ring, because there is much more light out here."*

Who is this person? What does weight-related success look like for them? What will motivate this individual to exert constructive focus on their weight and health for their lifetime? All of us, at times, hesitate to look beyond the superficial for answers. The search may be long, and the answers complex. Concentrating on the pounds gained; pointing out the unhealthy numerics; simplifying weight loss to "calories in, calories out"; or, ignoring the weight gain altogether—this overture feels manageable.

At least, such "answers" fit into a 15-minute appointment. Historically, however, this approach has led to high attrition, poor compliance, and poor outcomes. To look for the ring in the dark corners is the challenge that healthcare professionals face. The answers are not always obvious. On many days, healthcare professionals may doubt whether the person in front of them can really change. In fact, it's all too easy to grow weary of the seeming enormity of it all.

Accordingly, it's relatively easy to put patients on the defensive: "Your weight has gone up 10 pounds in the last five months. Don't let it get out of control." It's rarely, if ever, the doctor's intent to harm the patient. For the patient, however, such statements may feel accusatory, critical, and antagonistic. Some will pull back and others may eventually give up. Instead of feeling accomplished for managing exercise and eating over the last many months and "only gaining 10," the individual now feels "warned" and "reprimanded." What was previously felt as an accomplishment (it could have been 50 pounds gained) is now labeled "not good enough" and "watch out."

A study conducted by the Obesity Coalition Council (OCC), The Obesity Society (TOS), and the pharmaceutical company Eisai found that 80 percent of patients who are obese feel unmotivated to change after a doctor's visit. Furthermore, more than 60 percent don't believe the doctor is on their side.

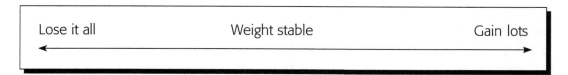

Lose it all   Weight stable   Gain lots

Healthcare providers may feel ill-equipped to travel down that haunted path, where patients describe having lost direction, motivation, and hope. As a consequence, the doctor's exam may have minimal focus on the origins of obesity, the contributing psychosocial factors, the patient's weight-related goals or interests, or the challenges related to weight management or weight loss.

A number of physicians may feel pressured by the conveyor belt of healthcare. Engaging a patient in a discussion about weight slows down a process that is typically rushed. In an article that appeared in Time magazine, "The Need for Better Obesity Education—In Medical Schools," a Harvard Medical school physician, Dr. James Colbert, opened up about this very problem:

> *Just seeing a patient walk into the clinic to see me, I can put them on a scale and measure their height and weight and calculate their body mass index and tell whether they are obese … But for me to figure out why that person is obese could take hours. And most physicians don't have that time.*

That situation could change, however. Following the AMA's classification of obesity as a disease, doctors anticipate increased medical reimbursement for obesity counseling. In other words, physicians will have more allowance to search for answers. In an article that asked doctors for their opinion on how classifying obesity as a disease will change their practice, one physician, Dr. Adam Goldstein, from University of North Carolina Family Medicine Center, said he looks forward to more time spent counseling obese patients:

> *We frequently squeeze [counseling] in, and we do it because it's the right thing to do … We need to drastically increase the reimbursement for counseling, and that will be true for obesity as much as it is for smoking cessation. The data suggest when we have these conversations, they're effective.*

For an epidemic that has seen relatively little effective positive change, the conversation with patients is where it can start.

EACH A UNIQUE STORY

Weight-related success is not just a number. The challenge is to identify what success looks like for each individual. No boilerplate exists. For some, slowing rapidly escalating weight may mean success. For others, weight stability may engender feelings of accomplishment. For still others, weight loss may not only be desired, but also possible.

Each person has a unique story. Accordingly, treatment decisions and/or weight-related advising must be tailored to meet the interests of each individual. The National Institutes of Health (NIH), one of the world's leading medical research centers, confirmed this in their report, published over a decade and a half ago:

> Standard treatment approaches for overweight and obesity must be tailored to the needs of various patients or patient groups. Large individual variation exists within any social or cultural group; furthermore, substantial overlap among subcultures occurs within the larger society. There is, therefore, no "cookbook" or standardized set of rules to optimize weight reduction with a given type of patient. However, to be more culturally sensitive and to incorporate patient characteristics in obesity treatment programs: consider and adapt the setting and staffing for the program; consider how the obesity treatment program integrates into other aspects of patient health care and self-care; and expect and allow for program modifications based on patient responses and preferences.

The patient's medical status is a priority. Patient interests are always first.

The whole person is the focus, not just numbers on the scale or BMI. If not numbers, then, what is a healthy weight?

WHAT CONSTITUTES HEALTHY?

A healthy weight is a maintainable weight. A healthy weight is one that an individual can maintain within the context of a balanced life. A healthy weight is one that leaves the individual with a reasonable sense of control. Healthy must be uniquely defined by each individual.

To lose hundreds of pounds—and maintain that weight for life—can be serious, time-consuming, and emotionally taxing. For most individuals, extreme weight loss demands a compulsive dedication to exercise, consume healthy food choices, and adhere to a level of commitment that can threaten their emotional wellness and life satisfaction. Who wants to wake up every morning of every day and feel ball-and-chained to a restrictive diet and an extreme exercise regime? In fact, most people will not sign on for a lifetime of exercise that feels punishing. However, a lifetime of carefully prescribed eating and daily rigorous exercise in preparation for extreme sports competition may be "fun" and rewarding for some individuals.

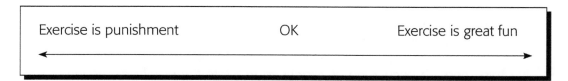

Extreme weight loss does not guarantee improved medical health. Weight loss does not promise weight-loss maintenance. Periods of weight loss may be followed by a lapse to disordered eating or the resumption of episodic binge eating. Some people can manage more weight change before reaching a threshold at which their weight runs (or ruins) their life and those relationships that give it meaning. Other individuals need to settle for less weight change.

Overshooting what's reasonable for the individual, based on pressure from the culture or what a chart says is ideal, often backfires. In reality, a stable weight is healthier than a cycling weight. Weight constantly in flux taxes both emotional and physical health. Repeated dieting and weight fluctuation may also be precursors for high blood pressure, high cholesterol, and slower metabolism, as well as plenty of frustration. In addition, a long history of "yo-yo" dieting can lead to the storage of fat around the middle section of the body, which increases a person's risk for diabetes, heart disease, stroke, high blood pressure, and even certain cancers.

Statistically, moderate weight loss, even just 10 percent of a person's weight, can lead to improved health. As the idea of "the fix" or the vision for "eliminating obesity" needs to be abandoned. The concept of "every single pound dropped and kept off forever" is likely an implausible feat for most individuals. Attempting to "take it all off" may actually further diminish good health. Accordingly, priority must be given to achieving a greater scientific understanding of the complexities of weight change, greater attention must be afforded to preserving weight stability, and greater credence placed on body, weight, and shape acceptance. Fundamental to preserving good health will be preventing unnecessary weight gain by adhering to reasonable amounts of physical activity, and a reasonable level of healthy eating, while avoiding extreme restrictive dieting and extreme weight loss.

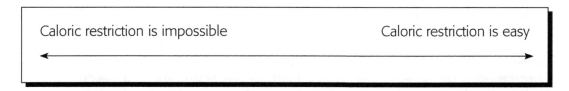

According to Joe Nadglowski, CEO and president of the Obesity Action Coalition (OAC), the results of a survey conducted by OAC reveal the need for an overhaul of the way obesity is treated:

> *We need to educate patients to have the conversation about their weight and ask the right questions so they leave the doctor's office feeling empowered to take steps toward managing their weight. We also need to encourage physicians to facilitate the weight discussion with their patients, as it is often a difficult topic to discuss.*

Arguably, overweight individuals don't need to be reprimanded or shamed. Patients desperately need an ally.

THE POWER OF ALIGNMENT

In only a few brief minutes, healthcare professionals attempt the impossible: listen in such a way that all patients leave the visit ready to take the next step to improve their health. To align with patients is to meet them where they are, not where they, the healthcare professionals, want them to be. It means withholding assumption and judgment. It means seeing each patient, their health condition, and related life circumstances through the patient's eyes, rather than broadly categorizing the individual as just another unmotivated "fat" person. When patients feel heard, as well as understood and respected, they are more likely to engage in a conversation about their health and feel motivated to protect their health.

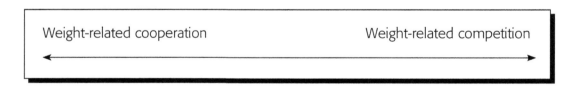

Weight-related cooperation   Weight-related competition

Physicians commonly assess the patient's potential health risk, share this information with the patient, and make treatment recommendations. Less common is the healthcare provider's assessment of the patient's readiness to change. Does the patient want to change their eating behavior or exercise patterns? Does the patient have any interest in weight change? Honestly, how does the patient really feel about the doctor's treatment recommendations?

In reality, the healthcare provider who is able to encourage the individual patient to express their own health-related interests and weight-related goals is a relatively uncommon occurrence. In the current medical-care environment, a patient is more likely to withhold their personal opinions about weight-related matters, avoid disagreeing with the medical advice, and/or tell the physician what they believe the physician wants to hear.

It doesn't take large amounts of weight loss to make big leaps forward toward improving a person's health. According to George Bray, MD, Ph.D., losing 5 percent of initial body weight can reduce the risk of developing diabetes, while a 5 to 15 percent weight loss from initial body weight can reduce most risk factors associated with dyslipidemia, hypertension, and diabetes mellitus.

Physicians who want to have a conversation with their patients about their interests and weight-related goals might consider the following foundational questions:

- What brings you to the office today?
- How would you like me to help you?
- What questions or concerns do you have about your health?
- How have your healthcare providers in the past been most helpful to you?
- Tell me about your health-related concerns or goals and how you are feeling about your recent progress.

"The more we hear them," according to Marshall Rosenberg, noted American psychologist, "the more they will hear us." To ask more open-ended questions ("How do you feel about your health?" and "What have you tried to do in the past to take care of yourself and how is that going for you?" and "How can I help you today?") is to look for the ring in the dark corners, where the answers aren't always so simple or obvious.

All factors considered, patients and families who feel heard are less defensive and more open to suggestion. This kind of communication aligns patient and healthcare worker in a way that enables them to better focus on the goal of improved health for the patient.

The approach should be empathic, collaborative, and genuine. The approach should be grounded in the desire to unearth the motivation that lies within every patient. This approach is similar to Motivational Interviewing (MI), which is employed in a variety of therapeutic settings (including smoking cessation, oral health, HIV risk reduction, alcohol addiction, and cancer prevention). MI has also been used effectively by healthcare providers in treating obesity.

A growing body of evidence shows that healthcare professionals can help patients become healthier simply by offering fewer instructions and asking more questions. MI is grounded in a number of assumptions. Change happens in small steps; relapse or lapse is normal; motivation is best considered on a continuum; and motivation is based on a patient's values. The underlying concept of MI is the principle that patients are more likely to discuss change and create action plans for change when asked what is important to them, rather than being lectured or told what is important. In their book, *How to Talk So Kids Can Learn*, authors Adele Faber and Elaine Mazlish write, "By teaching them how to approach a problem, by showing them how to break it down into manageable parts, by encouraging them to use their ingenuity to resolve their problems, we are giving them skills they can depend on for the rest of their lives.

That factor is true for children and adults. When people are invited to join us in tackling a problem, a powerful set of messages is sent: I believe in you. I trust your ability. I believe you can be wise. I believe you can be creative. I value your contributions in this process. I see our relationship as not all powerful, exercising authority over you, but as partners in mutually agreed upon pursuits. Not incompetence, not inexperience, but in equal dignity.

By teaching patients how to approach eating, weight, exercise, and health, healthcare professionals are not simply saying, "Here's how you fix it." They explore internal motivations. They empower growth that will be an ongoing resource for all pursuits as the experts in learning what will work for them. Patients are the experts in terms of their lives—which foods, activity, and relationships will best suit them and support their good health. The whole person, including their thoughts and feelings about personal health, is engaged in generating solutions and a viable course of action.

MI strategies presuppose that the patient's perspective is worth hearing. By acknowledging the patient's thoughts, circumstances, and emotions, a healthcare professional reduces the level of defensiveness experienced by the patient and opens the door to further collaborative discussions about weight-related matters. In addition, it creates space for the patient to self-observe, gain insight, and make connections that will be useful in implementing change after leaving the examination room. Among the steps that facilitate the healthcare professional in aligning with the patient are the following:

- Acknowledge that any change can be challenging or difficult.
- Encourage small and manageable goals.
- Clarify points of anticipated difficulty.
- Identify and discuss the primary emotions and thoughts that impede positive change.
- Reassure the patient and family that ambivalence is common and expected.

Allowing patients to simply speak frankly and openly about their ambivalence can be enormously helpful. Patients will leave feeling understood, respected, and better able to face challenge. A frank and calm discussion can facilitate desired behavior change.

THROUGH THE RESISTANCE

Resistance is to be expected. It comes in all forms, active and passive. The challenge is to learn the specifics of the patient's resistance, finding ways to respect that resistance, as well as to communicate that respect to the patient. Healthcare professionals have a number of actions they can undertake, when facing resistance, including the following:

- Acknowledge the patient's emotional state.
- Thoroughly hear the pros and cons of decisions regarding potential change.

- Discuss short- and long-term consequences of a behavior change.
- Delay agreeing or disagreeing with the patient's perspective. Hear the patient's perspective first.
- Be reminded that the patient will have great difficulty hearing the healthcare provider's opinions if the patient does not feel heard or understood.
- Avoid argument.
- Avoid the urge to win the argument or to prove the patient is wrong, at all costs. Consider carefully what you might be winning or losing.
- Prioritize the patient's personal health-related concerns and goals, whenever possible.

Emphasize the importance of the patients' rights and ability to make choices for themselves (as age-appropriate). The very moment when resistance appears may be the moment that leads to the greatest beneficial change. Whenever possible, summarize what you hear from the patient and/or their family.

- Here is what I heard you say about …
- I appreciated hearing more about …
- It sounds like you understand the benefits of _____ but that you also value _____.
- I am happy to talk with you more about _____.
- So, given what we talked about today, how would you like to proceed?

The result will be alignment—you and the patient, or you and the family. Furthermore, the result will be everyone working toward the same goal—improved health.

READING BETWEEN THE LINES

Communicating with patients about weight is fraught with possible missteps. It's easy to make wrong assumptions. A 300-pound person may recently have lost 50 pounds or gained 50 pounds or remained at the same weight for years. They might be an NFL linebacker or a teenager with a severe binge-eating disorder. While the number is the same in each situation, the circumstances differ vastly. The individual may or may not be knowledgeable in the principles of exercise and nutrition. As a result, the details of the patient's specific experience of their weight history will highlight their potential health risks and frustrations, as well as their degree of interest in advice or support.

Importantly, not all patients who make an appointment with their physician do so for the purpose of addressing symptoms related to weight. In fact, patients will often seek treatment for health concerns that are unrelated to their weight. Maybe a patient contracted strep throat from their grade school-age child, broke their toe while doing yard work, or woke with shooting pain in their rotator cuff.

Doctors who are particularly disdainful of overweight conditions may blame a person's excess weight for everything, from a stubbed toe to a respiratory infection to kidney failure. Forcing patients to step on a scale or lecturing them about their weight, when they are actually visiting for an eye infection, not only is not respectful, it may also disrupt patient-doctor communication in general and discourage future attendance for health-related appointments.

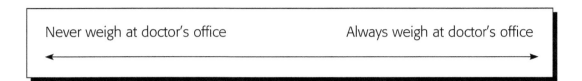

Never weigh at doctor's office   Always weigh at doctor's office

This point is illustrated by the following scenario in which a patient who seeks treatment for her seasonal allergies, is only to be asked, "Have you considered gastric bypass surgery? I can refer you to a bariatric surgeon." That situation is eregious. Unnecessary focus on weight and/or weighing may leave the patient feeling that their primary concern has been ignored or disrespected. Misattribution, known to occur when a doctor wrongly attributes a symptom to obesity, whittles away the trust that is essential to a doctor-patient relationship.

Dismissed, some patients give up on medical visits altogether, or delay their appointment until it's too late. This situation can lead to dire consequences. A friend told me the story of her sister who died of a treatable cancer because she stopped going to the doctor for five years after she was criticized for being too fat.

Discernment is critical. If weight is discussed before the patient's primary concern has been addressed, the doctor risks hijacking the appointment. While the physician may feel the patient's weight needs to be addressed, the primary purpose of the appointment should be respected. Patients appreciate being asked what they want from the appointment. Those concerns should be the priority unless there is a medical emergency.

Once the primary concerns have been addressed, healthcare providers can inquire further, for example, "Is there anything else I can help you with today? And, I see you are due for your yearly check-up soon. I will look forward to seeing you then." In an annual check-up, where the patient's overall health is being assessed, a physician could observe, "You didn't mention weight today. Do you have any concerns that I can help you address?" Or, "How are you feeling about your weight?"

Test results or positive findings that are weight-related should be inserted in the conversation simply and directly. It can be helpful to inquire how much the patient already knows or wants to know about the possible topics to be discussed. For example, "I know you stopped in today so we could take care of your eye infection, but, when I saw you last, you said you were interested in learning more about exercise. Would you like to talk more about that now?"

Attending to health-risk prevention is recommended. When possible and appropriate, the healthcare provider can focus on discussing modification of behaviors that contribute to weight-related conditions. In that regard, for example, doctors and patients can identify and measure behaviors, such as consuming high-sugar drinks, eating fruits and vegetables, engaging in minutes of enjoyable physical activity, attending meals with the family, and partaking of foods prepared at home. They can also discuss participating in activities that can contribute to good health, such as reducing screen time, walking to school, using stair steps, walking the dog, engaging in physically active recreational activities, and working in the yard or garden.

It is helpful to remember that body weight and numbers on a scale are not behaviors. Accordingly, numbers alone should not serve as targets of change.

Children, like adults, may fear that "weight talk" means that they are not doing something well enough, that they have not tried hard enough, and that they are "too fat." Children, like adults, will worry that someone will soon tell them to change their bodyweight or start dieting. They may fear that they will be required to give up their favorite or preferred foods. Furthermore, restriction of some favorite foods can increase the frequency of overeating and binge behavior.

If children or adults feel criticized about weight and shape, they may undertake a highly restrictive eating plan or engage in risky or extreme dieting practices that lower weight quickly, but in an unhealthy manner that may not be sustainable. Doctors who can inquire about the following factors before offering any specific feedback about weight may feel more aligned with their patients. Ultimately, they may also be more successful in supporting their patients' self-care:

- How physically active are you daily (in minutes or hours)?
- Do you like to exercise?
- How much screen time do you have daily—computer, phone, television, movies, etc. (in minutes or hours)?
- How are you doing with daily servings of fruit, vegetables, protein, and dairy?
- Are you able to eat slowly (e.g., mindfully)?
- Are you able to sit down for three meals and two snacks every day? (number of eating episodes)
- How is your sleep (in hours)?
- Do you wake feeling rested?
- How is your energy, mood, and focus during the day?
- How much stress do you experience daily (on an ascending scale of 1 to 10)
- What helps you manage your stress?
- What kinds of things have you been doing to take care of your health?

- In terms of your health, would you like to be doing anything differently?
- What prevents you from taking good care of yourself sometimes?
- Can I help you with any health-related concerns you might have?
- How are you feeling about your body weight or shape?
- Would you like my help in managing your concerns?

Weight alone never tells the whole story. Weight, BMI, and body composition information, however, can also be useful to track health trends that occur over time. As such, this information can be useful for professionals in the medical community in knowing how to accurately make health-related decisions, such as determining the proper dosage for prescribed medication.

Discussing weight-related numbers with the patient, without the discussion occurring as part of a larger consideration of the whole health picture, may have limited success and may, in fact, be detrimental.

Numbers-related feedback, in ideal terms, would simply provide information about an individual's personal health status and would motivate continued healthy self-care. This would be great news. Numbers-related feedback, however, can also prompt more body- and weight-related self-evaluation, self-criticism, and body-related obsessing. A numbers focus sometimes prompts risky practices, such as comparing oneself with others, engaging in restrictive eating, and/or beginning the next weight-loss plan. Unfortunately, the numbers discussion does not always bring the promise of better health.

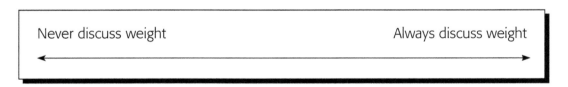

Feeling labeled, judged, or criticized can lead to subsequent weight gain, as opposed to weight loss. Unfortunately, words in the current culture, such as "fat," "obese," "overweight," "heavy," etc., typically have negative undertones, and are quickly associated with negative or unattractive personal qualities. Labeling the patient "obese" or classifying them as "overweight" may therefore result in the patient feeling criticized or frustrated. Lower self-esteem and/or mood may result with unhealthy eating behavior and possibly weight gain soon to follow.

It is beneficial for body weight to be considered as one component of the larger picture of overall health. On the other hand, since an individual's weight is determined by a large number of factors, caution should be exercised by healthcare providers with regard to any tendency to blame the patient for their overweight condition. It is also recommended that healthcare providers avoid any attribution of internal causality, such as, lazy, not trying hard enough, or just not knowing the right way to eat, etc. These attributions do not motivate improved health-related behavior or care.

Healthcare providers who lead their practice or clinic have a powerful opportunity to shape the positive attitudes of the people who toil in their workplace. There should be no tolerance for assigning blame in patient communication. The greater goal will be to help establish a "recovery culture," i.e., creating a safe place for patients, one in which only respectful, non- biased language is allowed.

According to Dr. Steve Harrington, Founder and Director of the National Association of Peer Specialists, "A recovery culture is founded on basic respect for individuals, served by mental health systems and self-respect on the part of clients themselves."

Such a culture requires that the entire team (from the receptionist to the doctor or therapist) adopt a holistic perspective on health, attend thoughtfully and compassionately to serving individuals of all sizes, and abstain from discriminatory language and behavior. Creating and maintaining a recovery culture will require ongoing and collaborative efforts of all administrative staff and healthcare providers. Concurrently, this group of professionals will need to attend to such considerations as they apply to the entire spectrum of healthcare: prevention, intervention, and recovery.

UNDERSTANDING MOTIVATION

Just because patients appear unmotivated to change doesn't mean that they don't want to change. As a rule, for every desire a person has, there is an opposing desire. In research involving individuals with eating disorders, Dr. Steven Stern, a Portland- and University of Maine-based psychologist, notes the importance of the "management of contradictory, opposing currents." In other words, for all people, there are simultaneously occurring and competing motivations for change.

For example, people may be motivated to both wake up early in the morning to tackle school or work projects and motivated to sleep longer, because they feel tired and want more sleep. Children may be motivated to eat vegetables because they understand that they are good for their health, and simultaneously motivated to avoid eating vegetables, because they find the taste to be undesirable. Motivations to change behavior may be more unidirectionally aligned in an emergency or critical event. Firefighters, for example, are motivated to protect both themselves and other people. In an emergency, their motivation to serve others may take priority.

The healthcare provider may at times view their patient as "unmotivated" to better manage weight-related behavior. This assumption, however, may be based on some information, but not all of the information. In most life moments, there exists various co-occurring and competing motivations. In other words, there are reasons to change behavior, as well as reasons to not change behavior that exist simultaneously.

Healthcare professionals who are able to investigate further for evidence of motivation to change eating or exercise behavior can learn more about how best to help the patient they are treating. For example, they might learn that the patient is willing to walk more frequently but is recovering from an ankle injury and wants to give it more rest time to heal. They could learn that the patient is wanting to make healthy food choices for themselves and their family but also wants to live within a relatively small food budget. Furthermore, the healthcare professional might learn that the patient is attempting to curb caloric intake to reduce weight, but also wants to quell the consequential increased hunger pangs and low energy. Having a discussion to clarify awareness of an individual's competing motivations may actually facilitate that patient's progress.

Other factors known to motivate weight-related behavior change include supportive family or friends, the ability to adhere to enjoyable physical activity, reasonable expectations, and belief in the ability to change. Motivation is highest when interest in achievement originates within the individual. Attribution theory warns of the dangers of other people (e.g., parents, friends, culture, and healthcare providers) pushing behavioral change. Powerful external motivators can decrease internal motivation. Motivation is highest when personal values and interest drive the elected change.

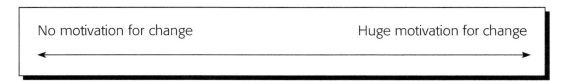

Healthcare providers can have a meaningful impact on informing and supporting their patient's health. Some patients have never felt hopeful enough to even fully consider what lasting change entails. Other patients feel that they aren't equipped with the necessary skills to identify and clarify their personal motivation for change. Healthcare providers can support individuals in finding their own interests and goals.

In fact, healthcare providers, who prescribe the ideal or advise a specific fix, risk imposing their own cultural version of health (e.g., the thin ideal) onto the patient. To do so means that healthcare providers have implicitly aligned themselves with the proposition that assumes the obese patient needs to lose a certain amount of weight. The real challenge, however, is to align medical support with the patient's preferred interests and goals.

For some patients, the goal is simply to achieve weight stability. Other patients may be interested in weight change. In that situation, the focus of change must target behavior, as opposed to numbers. Behaviors that are modified slowly and gradually are often more sustainable than those that involve sudden and dramatic change.

Weight change or weight loss may not be of interest to the patient. This perspective should be respected by the healthcare provider. For example, weight-related goals for this population may simply involve something like attaining greater personal self-awareness, improving personal self-control, gaining greater awareness of hunger cues, achieving improved control in eating, accomplishing greater comfort in exercising in public, and/or having more enjoyment in physical activity. As such, helping clients set realistic goals is critical not just for the patient's weight-related health, but for their self-esteem. Anticipating consequences and discussing them prior to effecting change is a great opportunity to plan ahead for how best to respond to potential setbacks.

Internationally renowned nutritional expert, Kelly D. Brownell, notes that while there is hardly any correlation between a person's actual physical attractiveness and their satisfaction with their body image, there is a correlation between body image and self-esteem. Ultimately, it's about helping patients take control of their health, rather than have their health more solely controlled by magazine covers and weight loss advertisements. All factors considered, the healthcare provider and the patient will find greater short-term and longer-term success if they are aligned in understanding the personal goals of their patient and are united in how to address any related change.

The underlying hope is that rather than attempting to "fix" the "weight problem," healthcare professionals might learn more about prevention, more about new perspectives and definitions of weight-related success, and more about understanding and supporting the interests of their patients. Defining weight as the problem misses both the problem and the fix. When possible, healthcare providers should step away from the numbers and become a greater resource for providing sound information and helping the patient progress toward achieving agreed-upon and identified goals.

Obesity will never be eliminated. Obesity itself is not the problem. Obesity is the symptom of greater culture-wide problems. If obesity, as is pointed out in Chapter 2, is never the result of "just one thing," then it must be addressed in multiple ways with recognition that obesity is one symptom, but not one condition.

Obviously, healthcare professionals cannot provide all the answers to the issue of obesity. Physicians, registered dieticians, psychologists, sociologists, or exercise physiologists cannot curb the obesity trends alone. Furthermore, teachers, policymakers, and community leaders cannot act alone to effect the needed changes. In fact, individuals acting alone are not capable of making the necessary changes to the amalgam of systems that have perpetuated obesity for decades.

Americans turn to physicians when questions about health-related goals arise. They always have. On the other hand, no one should count on doctors to solve weight and weight-related issues by themselves. When physicians feel hopeless about their patient's condition, they will call "hospice." Healthcare providers must not give up. They must take the extra time to learn, as well as to look for the less-than-easy answers and serve as the conduit for all of the available resources that can help solve the problems. Healthcare professionals and treatment providers must leave "no one behind." Individuals of all sizes deserve respect and excellent healthcare. Unless ideas are integrated from multiple sources, and a collaborative and synchronized effort is created, obesity will continue to be perceived as a one-dimensional medical problem, with the impossible, one-dimensional medical fix.

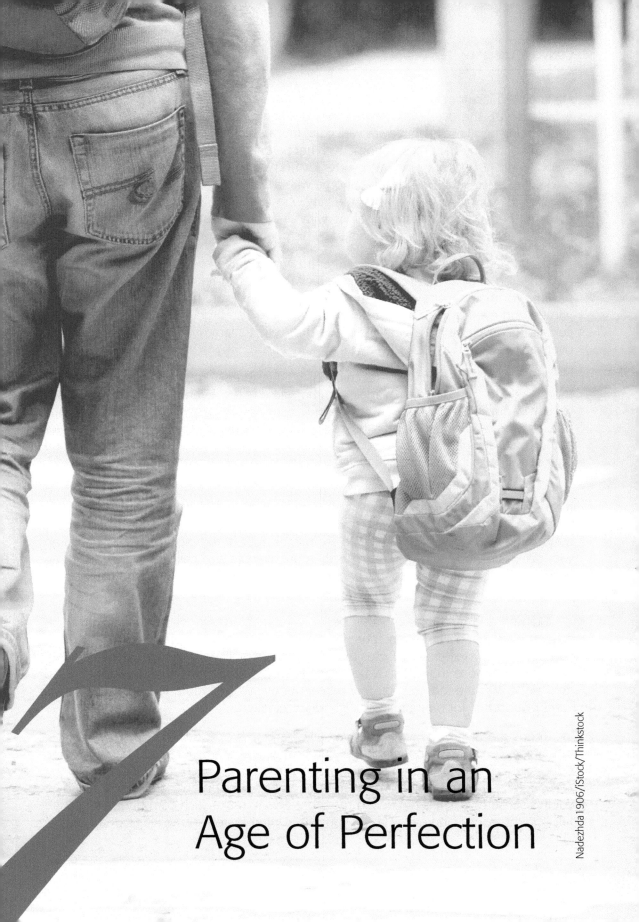

Parenting in an Age of Perfection

He is picked last for every game of kickball during recess. She eats alone at lunchtime. A table down, she overhears the thin girls, dressed in size-four cut-off shorts, complain about being fat. He says he may as well go to fat camp, while the rest of his troop attends the Jamboree. She hangs out at home with her parents, while her "bestie," and seemingly every other 16-year-old girl, has a date for homecoming. He pretends to ignore the snickering; he was the only one sent home with a "fat letter." She asks her parents if she can skip school on occasion, facing the girls who called her "fat and ugly" on Facebook the night before is too much. He, along with all the other out-of-shape ninth-graders, is relegated to the lower gym class, coined by his peers as fat gym.

As fat hatred bleeds into the culture, it is no surprise overweight children and, in fact, children of all sizes, are discriminated against. Weight-related bullying of peers is a pastime for many youth, who learn the vice from television, movies, magazines, video games, and even by well-intended parents, who are also products of the weight-biased culture. Research paints a grim picture of the weight stigma affecting the one-in-three overweight children in the U.S.

One study found that obese children, grades three through six, are 65 percent more likely to be bullied than their slimmer classmates. Even if the child possesses winsome qualities, like being a good student or having a great personality, bullying persists. The lead researcher for the study, Julie Lumeng, M.D., professor of pediatrics at the University of Michigan, reported, "What we found is that ... no matter how good your social skills, if you were overweight or obese, you were more likely to be bullied."

In American culture, fat is predominantly unlikeable. In 2003, researchers replicated a study conducted during the early 1960s that instructed more than 600 10- to 11-year-old kids to view six pictures of children and rank them in order of with whom they would want to be friends. Of the six images, four of the pictures were of children with disabilities, one was of a perceivably more-average size child, and one was of an obese child. Then, as well as now, the image of the obese child was liked the least. In fact, over 50 years later, the aversion grew by over 40 percent.

Bullying and discrimination that begin in elementary school persist into the high school years, often with even more cruelty. Sixty-four percent of weight-loss seeking youth said they experienced weight-bullying at school. Perhaps the most haunting reality is that those individuals who were perceived as friends laughed and ridiculed right along with the masses. Seventy percent of overweight youth reported that friends were responsible for perpetrating weight discrimination.

Teens are physically, as well as verbally, harassed; excluded from social activities; the targets of fat jokes; the grist of the rumor mill, and the recipients of hateful phone calls, texts, emails, and comments on social media. As such, a "selfie" posted on Facebook, Instagram, Twitter, Tumbler, or any other social media outlet can destroy a youth's sense of self. It is not uncommon for peers to make such comments as, "you're fat," "go throw up," and even "go kill yourself." Unfortunately, some kids try and do so.

Ally Del Monte, a 15-year-old blogger, chronicles in a blog the torture of being bullied because of her weight. For a two-year period, peers (girls whom she once called friends), shunned her, participating in the "don't talk to Ally days" at school. Other days, peers slammed her into lockers, spit on her, and isolated her at lunch time, telling her to throw up her meal. Repeatedly, she was told she was fat, worthless, disgusting, and that she should go kill herself. "Why can't you fall down the stairs and break your neck?" or "Your mom should have aborted you!" her peers told her.

When students accessed her private "Tumblr account," and she received 270 emails in one night telling her to kill herself, she despaired. Ally states, "I started to believe it. I wanted to die." So, she found a bottle of Advil and her dad's heart medication, and was determined to end her life. While Ally's story has a happy ending (her mom heard the bottle of pills drop in the bathroom), there are countless untold stories of youth whose stories don't.

This situation is the den of lions into which children at any weight are tossed and must battle to survive. This is the environment where perpetrators of discrimination act and others join in or turn away. All children are surrounded by labeling, blaming, shaming, and hurt. There are no winners.

The effort to survive is exacerbated in the private sector, whereby relatively few efforts have been made to contain the floodwaters of obesity. After all, the food industry, built on the production of junk food and processed foods that fuel humans' addictions to these foods, stands to lose billions of dollars of market share. Recently, the food industry, led by name-brand juggernauts like Burger King, General Foods, and the Coca-Cola Company, appeared to be laying sandbags when it launched the Children's Food and Beverage Advertising initiative, which is designed to encourage marketing of healthier dietary choices and a healthy lifestyle to children under 12.

Not much has changed, however. In fact, it might even be worse. In her article that appeared in the July 2012 *PLOS Medicine* journal, "Thinking Forward: The Quicksand of Appeasing the Food Industry," internationally renowned expert on obesity, Kelly Brownell, writes that "objective reports ... have shown a tidal wave of marketing of calorie-dense, nutrient-poor foods to children, and if any change is occurring, marketing is on the increase." To become a partner in the battle against obesity, the implicit demand of the food industry is to sell less of their more profitable food. It seems such a demand is too high a cost for organizations that are part of this industry.

Not too long ago, Coca-Cola launched an obesity-awareness campaign, the irony of which was too obvious not to pan. The situation involved a global brand trying to apologize for how it makes money. Does Coca-Cola move out of the bottling and distribution business? Not at all. Over the past few years, Coke has been acquiring various brands of beverages, from water to juices to even coconut beverages in anticipation of a significant drop in soda consumption. Accordingly, when challenged by the government and medical communities regarding their products, they reply that they offer a spectrum of choices for the individual.

Seven percent of calories of our collective diet come from soda, reports Mark Bittman, writer on food for the *New York Times* and author of the *VB6* and *The VB6 Cookbook*. Furthermore, as Bittman states, "So, it's up to us to remember that Coke makes its money selling sugar-sweetened beverages, and even when they're apologizing for that, as they appear to be doing here—they're still selling them."

It's not that Coca-Cola is apologizing for their products and tremendous skill at the distribution of beverages all over the world, it's that they see the trend today and have been preparing for the future where they can maintain the competitive advantage of bottling and product distribution to all parts of the globe. While their strategy will allow the individual to make the choice that is best for them, the array of options is essentially dominated by products bottled by Coca-Cola.

Coca-Cola is in the selling business … and sell they do. Coca-Cola's Facebook page had 100 million youth visitors in 2015. Twenty-one sugary drink brands had YouTube channels in 2015, with collectively 7.2 million users and over one billion views by Oct 2016.

As children grow into adults (and most grow even larger), the discrimination continues, though it may manifest itself differently. For example, in the workforce, overweight individuals, when stacked against their slimmer counterparts, are denied jobs, overlooked for promotions, and deprived of raises. Born out of the stereotype that "lazy" and "unmotivated" are a measure of a person's extra weight, overweight individuals are perceived as neither powerful nor in control.

Individuals need to look no further than the pre-2016 presidential election landscape for an affirmation of the existence of such an attitude. In February 2013, New Jersey Governor and presidential hopeful Chris Christie underwent lap band surgery to whittle away the girth that belied his power. In a similar vein, parents, who realize that success is linked to thin, often hold their breath as their obese child faces their first interview. In reality, the obese individual may indeed be crushed by rejection, just like they were as a child. This time, however, who will provide the obese person with a soft landing?

Parents spend wakeless nights imagining their overweight child alone as an adult. One recent study by a Swedish researcher found that men who by the age of 18 are grossly overweight were nearly 50 percent less likely to be married in their 30s and 40s than their "normal" counterparts. Another study determined that courting is largely based on appearance and a culturally acceptable weight.

A Columbia University economist, Pierre-Andre Chiappori, and his colleagues wrote an article titled "Fatter Attraction," in which they reviewed a formula that they developed that shows how men and women who have a higher BMI can enhance their chances of finding a spouse in the marriage market. According to their research, appearance is the primary currency in the marriage market, though an overweight man can enhance his marketability if his work wage is higher and a heavier woman can compensate with extra education.

The irony of the situation, however, is that overweight individuals don't typically (or quickly) climb the corporate ladder. Furthermore, obese teenage girls are less likely than their thin counterparts to enroll in college, especially when obesity is not the norm at their institution. The message is that weight bias exists—a level of prejudice that all too often serves as a barrier to success.

THE PROBLEM WITH PERFECTION

Parents may fear the collateral effect of their child's weight or appearance, an attribute that may cause more harm than good. Fear drives a parent to unknowingly shame their child—"You'd look better if you lost 50 pounds." To compare their child—"Look at John. He looks so muscular. He must exercise a lot more than you do." To restrict their child—"No more TV, until you drop 10 pounds." To bargain with their child—"If you drop 15 pounds and prove to me you care about your appearance, then you can get braces." Or, "Lose all the weight, and we will buy you a puppy." As a result, the endless dieting cycle is perpetuated—"The doctor says your weight is too high; you need to start a diet." Unfortunately, these strategies further aggravate the problems.

It can be helpful to keep in mind the fact that children do not elect to live in an "obesiogenic" environment, surrounded by calorie-dense foods and having little need for physically active living. A child doesn't choose his genetics, a factor that is often more responsible for the development of obese conditions than many of the other determinants combined. He doesn't choose his family environment, which may not value sport or recreation or have the knowledge base to understand the health benefits of eating nutritionally balanced meals.

Our children do not choose the neighborhoods in which they live, which may be a food desert and/or lacking parks or recreation centers. He doesn't choose his schools, which may not offer physical education and healthy meals. For a number of recent years, the most physical exertion on a typical day at most schools has involved carrying a backpack full of books. This situation has dramatically changed. Textbooks have been replaced with "iPads," "lap-tops," or other hand-held electronic devices. While scrolling and texting are increasingly popular pastimes, they are not known for high levels of caloric expenditure or improved cardiovascular health.

The sad truth is that many children would need to overcome innumerable environmental conditions to maintain good health and inevitably will wind up feeling punished for not being able to change the unchangeable. Not surprisingly, children, whose bodies are not infinitely malleable, are frustrated by inflexible standards, often imposed within highly obesiogenic environments.

Obesity is rarely about just one factor, e.g., "willpower." Parents may look at their neighbor's "skinny" or alleged "perfect child" and believe that with the right amount of effort their child could or should look like that. The truth, however, is that kids come in different shapes and sizes, dissimilarities that are often determined by genetics. When a parent declares that their child's shape is a problem, that attitude is often soon re-interpreted as "the child is the problem." Feeling alone, out of control, and "not good enough," many children turn to food behaviors, such as over-restriction or binge eating, to cope. As a consequence, the weight cycle continues.

Many parents want to be helpful and support their children's health. They may, however, lack empathy for the enormous effort it takes to survive in a body that doesn't fit in with the current culture's expectations. Fearing for their child's future, they may feel compelled to communicate or behave in ways that are emotionally hurtful. For example, some parents may assume their son doesn't care about his weight, because he hasn't lost any weight.

It can be far too easy for parents to jump to conclusions when their 13-year-old son is sitting in front of the TV, with bags of chips and juice boxes strewn about the floor. "Doesn't he realize what he is doing to himself?" As a result, the parents may step in with misdirected comments, such as "Do you know how many calories are in those juice boxes? With the chips and juice, you've already consumed half of your daily recommended caloric intake!"

It's not easy parenting in an age of perfection. It's the student who scores a 36 on the ACT, the all-star jock, the right zip code, the enviable title, and the homecoming queen whom culture believes have the most promise. According to the popular cultural perspective, to have a chubby child with a 3.0 GPA is to lead a life of invisible mediocrity.

Too many individuals believe that success has much more to do with the array of boundless measurable and observable externals, than what's on the inside of a person. It is a fact of life that values, personal interests, and character receive much less press. The cultural pull for perfection is an insurmountable force. It's the underlying bankrupt promise of the thin ideal.

The pressure to attain and maintain perfection can lead to anxiety, depression, addictions, eating disorders, and, even, suicide. Perfection doesn't allow for human error. It also does not permit time and space for learning and personal growth to occur. The pursuit of perfection may promise rewards, but actually disrupts performance, increases frustration, adds stress, and zaps motivation for sustained health-related efforts.

If someone hands a football to a kid who never has played football and says, "Throw it 50 yards," he likely will not immediately succeed. He might conclude, "I can't throw." On the other hand, if someone hands the ball to him and says, "Give it a try," and he throws it five yards, he might conclude, "I did it." Given similar conditions, he may be motivated to try again and perhaps throw it six yards the next time.

In recognizing his effort and providing modest expectations for execution, the likelihood that the kid will be interested in learning to throw and perhaps continuing to pursue activity or sport may increase. Striving for excellence is different than striving for perfection. The first targets the process, while the latter concentrates on the results. If a parent expects perfection, their children will come up short. Similarly, if a parent tells their child to lose weight and get skinny, the message may be de-motivating or be interpreted as:

- "You are not good enough the way you currently are."
- "You are a disappointment to me."
- "You are acceptable, only if you change."
- "You don't understand that you are damaging your health."
- "Your efforts are not enough."
- "Your accomplishments are recognizable, only when you have reached a pre-defined and ideal outcome."

A young man whose family was one of Chicago's elite was 250 pounds. His parents hobnobbed with the mayor, millionaires, and megastars. On an almost daily basis, he had what might have appeared to be "perfection" paraded in front of him. He struggled to keep up with the expectations regarding his image. After dedicating himself to healthier eating and finding his way to enjoyable physical activities, he dropped to 215 pounds. For several years, he maintained that weight, improved his health, and contributed profitably to his family's business.

Periodically, I see his parents, and they ask, "When is he going to get down to 190 pounds?" "Just 25 pounds more to go," they declare. While the parents are loving and well-meaning, their sentiments suggest the hyper-focus on thin and sadly reverberate the message that "You're not good enough." *Why is "good" not "good enough?"*

Some parents seek perfection for their kids, because they believe it will bring happiness for themselves and for their children. Some parents believe that having *"perfect kids"* is proof of *"perfect parenting."* Other parents seek perfection because they fear judgment by the Joneses. This fear may drive "image" management. They agonize over what they think others think about their kids and their parenting: *My God, do they ever tell her no? Why don't they get her into an exercise program? Are they lazy?* To accept their child's less-than-perfect physique would be giving up or admitting that they are the "losers" and that the "Joneses win."

Learning to quiet the cultural noise that screams that their child is not good enough can be challenging. That noise surrounds them every day. Such cultural noise may also scream that they aren't good enough parents. Many parents may not easily accept their child's imperfections, in part because they have not yet accepted their own.

If the parents are still being critical of their own body, how can they adopt "mindful acceptance" when it comes to their kids? Mothers, especially, are guilty of "fat talk." Fat talk is the everyday negative statements about an individual's body that reinforce the thin ideal, e.g., "I look so fat in those jeans." "Look at my muffin top!" "That picture confirms that I need to drink only water for the next week."

In many ways, fat talk is a plea for affirmation in a world that doesn't recognize average. For a number of women, however, fat talk is the overflow of a woman's internal self-loathing. In a provocative blog post on the *Huffington Post* that went viral in 2013, "When Your Mother Says She's Fat," author Kasey Edwards candidly talked about how her mother's unrelenting fat talk tragically set the stage for her own struggle with self-hatred:

> *With every grimace at your reflection in the mirror, every new wonder diet that was going to change your life, and every guilty spoon of "Oh-I-really-shouldn't," I learned that women must be thin to be valid and worthy. Girls must go without because their greatest contribution to the world is their physical beauty. Just like you, I have spent my whole life feeling fat. When did fat become a feeling anyway? And because I believed I was fat, I knew I was no good.*

As parents grimace at their reflections, pursue the next miracle diet, and guiltily eat a spoonful of the forbidden, their children absorb the not-so-subtle message that "If I'm fat, then I'm no good." Studies show that children model parents' eating behavior and attitudes, which can either facilitate or impede a healthy attitude toward eating and weight. Arguably, a better parental example is that which Edwards calls for at the end of her piece:

> *"Let us honor and respect our bodies for what they do instead of despising them for how they appear. Focus on living healthy and active lives, let our weight fall where it may, and consign our body hatred in the past where it belongs."*

Unfortunately, most teens, especially girls, struggle to let their weight fall where it may. Weight gain for many adolescent girls is more terrifying than getting cancer, nuclear war, or losing their parents. To sit at home on prom night because you're the fat girl may feel like life is over. Not surprisingly, the thin ideal drives droves of pre-teens to dieting.

In 1970, the average age a girl started dieting was 14 years. By 1999, the average age dropped to eight years. In fact, recent studies estimate that 50 percent of fourth grade girls describe themselves as on a diet. The tragedy, however, is that the earlier the first dieting behavior presents itself in a lifetime, the greater the likelihood of an eating disorder and the more severe the obese condition. Unaware of the risky consequences, a number of loving parents push diets, knowing no other means to protect their children and curb the feared weight gain.

Unfortunately, contrary to popular belief, dieting behavior among adolescents is associated with weight gain and not weight loss. In fact, adolescent frequent dieters are seven times (boys) to 12 times (girls) more at risk for binge eating than non-dieters. In a recent study that I conducted with a colleague, we investigated the impact of restrictive parent-child feeding practices during childhood. Our research involved having male and female adult patients complete a brief questionnaire that assessed problems with binge eating, previous diagnosis of binge eating disorder, the presence of a diet mentality during childhood, and their parents' or caregivers' management of food, diet, and weight-related practices during their childhood. Specifically, participants were asked to examine the restrictive or punishing nature of their childhood parenting environment, as it related to food, including the availability of "enough" food in their childhood home; the presence or absence of food rules; restrictions related to calorically dense foods (e.g., desserts); the punishment for eating certain foods; the freedom granted to eat at any time; and any reactions to the restrictions (e.g., sneaking or hiding food, negative body image).

The study revealed that participants with a history of binge eating behaviors and participants with a prior binge eating disorder diagnosis experienced higher levels of restrictive parent-child feeding practices in comparison to participants without a history of binge eating or diagnosis. *Simply stated, restriction and/or punishment intended to control weight actually leads to more out-of-control eating and weight gain.* Why would that be?

A friend recently told me a story about a dinner party at which she observed a two-year-old sitting in a high chair for the duration of a three-hour meal. Yes, that's right—for three whole hours. Initially, my friend was impressed, remembering that her children, when they were young, would not tolerate that sort of lengthy confinement. The mother of the child achieved this parenting feat through bribery with food, lecturing, and scolding. Think about what the mother accomplished—obedience through external and primarily manipulative means. Yes, you can teach a two-year-old to sit in a high chair for three hours. Food is a powerful reinforcement. At what cost, however?

In this example, the parent wanted to dine and visit with friends for several hours. The child likely wanted to run around, play, and explore. The child might learn that their needs are less important than the parents,' and therefore the child is less important or less valued than other people. The child learns that the parents' interests or needs supersede their own. If the pattern repeats itself over the child's life, the child may become more vigilant of the needs of others and less able to be aware of their own needs, wants, and, yes, hunger. After all, what would be the point of an individual being *mindful* of their own needs, if there is no opportunity to work toward communicating those needs or having those needs met? Frustration is certain; depression, low self-esteem, and resentment are likely.

Similarly, while a parent can force their child to begin a diet, what might be the longer-term consequences of that action? Diets, traditionally understood, are an external imposition. When does the child determine what they really want, and who they want to be? The culture, or what is perceived as the norm in American culture, has specific ideas about how kids should behave and what they *should* achieve.

Obviously, it's good parenting to influence, educate, and appropriately discipline children. Some parents, however, impose control to the extent that it can interfere with healthy emotional development or, in some cases, "arrested social-emotional development." How does the child grow into who they are? Some children hit their teen and early adult years and don't know who they are or what they really want.

One of my teenage patients recently complained of severe depression, stating that she didn't even have the energy to do homework, plan for college, or even go to school. She explained that she currently had no motivation to get out of bed in the morning. When I asked her to tell me more about that she stated, "Why even try? My mother has hijacked my life. I would just be living her life and not my own."

Controlling children with food or cajoling them with rewards to produce a specific outcome does not necessarily instill personal values in them, help them discover their talents or passions, or ensure their ability to make good decisions when they are older. Well-intended, hard-working parents may unwittingly raise their children conditioned to be what others expect them to be, as opposed to be well-oriented to whom they truly are.

A person's emotional self is core to healthy adult functioning. Emotional awareness and constructive emotional expression are like the foundation of a house. It's hard to think about decorating a home whose foundation is crumbling or unstable. The next storm makes it vulnerable to collapse. Without a strong sense of their deepest emotions, needs, values, preferences, and passions (including the internal cues that help them determine if they're hungry, why they're hungry, what they're hungry for, and what will satisfy their hunger), individuals tend to default to how they have been conditioned to think.

Often, that condition is cultural and powerfully influenced by the ideals of "thin" or other extreme ideals. The person who finishes first is the winner, fastest, smartest, best. This mindset is why so many people fixate on a number. In the absence of clarity of identity, a black hole exists that may be filled by dieting thoughts, eating rules, body image frustrations, and numbers.

Fixating on weight-related numbers may feel easier than the experiences of a person knowing the "emptiness" of their emotional world. In fact, the more individuals are drawn away from paying attention to their emotional experience and who they uniquely are, the more they tend to crave the reward of the number. The diet (external truth) becomes the internal narrator of what a person is "supposed to do" or "should be." As a result, permission to be more natural themselves is withheld from that individual.

INTERNAL CONTROLS

If restrictions, rules, punishment, and getting skinny don't work, what, if anything, can parents do to support their children's health?

First, parents will benefit from realizing that there is no program that will create the perfect child. Perfection does not exist. Encouraging a child to embrace healthy choices is dependent upon the parent's "buy-in" to a counter-cultural way of thinking—one that says, "I love you as you are." "I do not expect you to change your weight." One that asks, "How can I support your health ?" or "How can I empower you to take good care of yourself?" "How can I help you enjoy physical activity?" or "How can I make healthy food choices easy for you?" One that inquires, "How can I help you become you?" One that accepts setbacks: "We all have those days." Or, "I want you to look like you, and to be you."

A study of individuals with longer-term anorexia found that women who had an eating disorder for an average of 15 years recovered when their treatment was focused on personal values, their unique interests, and their quality of life, as opposed to just "numbers." When treatment targeted weight, calories consumed, the scale, eating patterns, or improving their health, recovery was stalled. Similarly, parents might do better to help their children focus on developing relationships they enjoy, cultivating activities of interest, and leading lives they value, rather than relentlessly pursuing diets and weight-related targets.

Second, parents can learn to replace rigid rules with healthy modeling, as well as sound information and appropriate *"guidelines."* Younger children may benefit from more narrow decision-making parameters, while older children tend to respond better to more broad measures. Unlike the "good food and bad food" rules that proclaim, "You can't eat this," guidelines provide options within safe boundaries. Kids of all ages like to have some decision-making power. For example, younger children can choose between which fruit to have with their lunch or whether their preference is to go to a park to play on the swings or to ride their bikes. In turn, older kids can choose their sandwich or soup preference or which after-school sport or recreational activity to join.

The important point to remember is that everyone makes better food choices when they are not "starving." Creating an environment conducive to healthy eating means ensuring that one or two snacks daily and three meals per day are available every day. Neither a food lock-up nor a calorie free-for-all will work. The challenge is to create an environment in which the child will continue to recognize personal feelings of hunger and satiety, will enjoy eating well, will have permission to express food preferences, is encouraged to try new foods, and does not fear food or body-related criticism or punishment.

One of my clients once reported to me that she found candy wrappers underneath her child's bed. She was confounded. Martha Stewart couldn't produce a more balanced meal. She made sure that every meal was comprised of brown rice, vegetables, and a fist-size portion of protein. Even the snacks were locked up in a drawer.

Subsequently, I asked her to consider what the *"locked drawer of treats"* conveyed to her daughter. She struggled for an answer. Together, we considered several possibilities. For example, "You can't control healthy food choices without the lock;" "You cannot be trusted;" or "I expect that you will break the rules." After some discussion, we agreed that her daughter was learning that her parents could not trust her and perhaps worse, she could not even trust herself. These are messages that can linger for a lifetime and can impact a child's level of confidence and physical and emotional well-being, far into the future.

Several studies have found that parental restriction of a child's intake of palatable foods is associated with overconsumption of those foods when free access to those items is subsequently permitted. It's not surprising that college students are notorious for gaining the "freshman 15," under the newly discovered unsupervised and unrestricted food conditions. For many individuals, this situation is the first time that they have had such liberty in their food choices. Having a history of being confronted with rigid food rules, a fear of food-related punishment, a labeling of foods as good or bad, restricted access to food, or possibly the "treats being locked up" can contribute to loss of control when exposed to more independent decision-making.

Humans have hunger signals. When the parent takes complete control over how much the child eats, the child, in essence, loses the ability to rely on those signals. Instead of locking up the drawer, I encouraged the mom to put a variety of snacks in the drawer and make them available. The mom worried that her daughter would overeat. I agreed that while her daughter may do so, given her new access, I hoped that it would be for a brief time.

Subsequently I encouraged the mom to undertake several steps, including to minimize out-of-control hunger by frequently providing healthy snacks and meals; to avoid topics of conversation with her daughter that focus narrowly on weight or appearance-related matters; to avoid the use of food as a punishment or a reward for her daughter; to put the healthy snacks in readily available locations; to no longer require her daughter to eat everything on her plate; to model positive body-image communication; and to avoid discussions with her daughter that are focused on comparing body shape or size. In fact, locking up food may increase the desirability of that food. It was hoped that the recommended environmental modifications, over time, would permit her daughter to reduce any eating or food-related anxiety that she might have and to better self-regulate her eating by tuning into her own body's signals.

Such a concern is common among parents: If I don't lock up the potato chips, they'll eat the entire bag. I always respond by asking them to consider creating an environment in which that situation will be less likely to happen. Instead, they should offer a variety of healthy-snack options. What if when their children came home from school, they had carrot sticks, apple slices, cheese sticks, and ice water set out on the counter? Later on, when they make snack choices for themselves, they may be more apt to choose the healthier options.

Parents should consider placing the healthier food options at the front of the fridge. Another step might be to increase the frequency of eating so their child doesn't dip into starvation mode. If the child is going to be on the run all day, a cooler of snacks could be prepared so that the fast food isn't their stopgap. Forbidding desserts should be avoided. To deny their child dessert is only to intensify the craving for it.

Another option for a parent to consider is having the child help create meals that are healthy and enjoyable for the entire family, especially if the child is hesitant to try new foods. Smelling and tasting the food during preparation can pique an interest in an "I'll-never-try-it" food. Parents can also pack a lunch comprised of different food groups. While the package can include a dessert, it could also contain include fruit, vegetables, healthy grains, and a lean-protein item. While a parent's son or daughter may not eat it all every day, by making it, the parent is providing good options and healthy opportunities for their children.

It can also be very helpful for parents to check in with their kids about their lunch preferences and problem-solve together to identify food combinations that suit everyone's interests. It is important to be aware of the fact that if a child doesn't eat all of their lunch, so be it—let it go. It's not about perfection. It's a process.

THE POWER OF PLAY

The most effective obesity-related health programs address a combination of nutrition, behavior, physical activity, and parent involvement. Because obesity is multi-dimensional, it must be addressed from multiple angles. As such, lifestyle interventions that involve families have been determined to be the most effective for controlling weight.

In my office, families are encouraged to engage in activity together, e.g., go for a bike ride, walk to school, host a Wii "just dance" party, join a climbing class, garden, toss a Frisbee, go hunting, etc.—whatever is enjoyable and encourages body movement. Parents are not allowed to be physically inactive, while expecting their kids to be sport superstars. This approach simply does not work.

When a family goes on vacation, destinations should be sought that provide opportunities for activity, like paths on which to bicycle, a pool in which to swim, rivers in which to fish, trails on which to hike, etc. When possible, create an environment for play and activity. It is also about developing a set of values about activity within the family. For example, activity is enjoyable; activity draws the family together; activity helps to relieve stress; activity clears the head; and activity increases self-confidence and awareness.

To frame activity as enjoyable, rather than punishing, will help encourage a child to seek it out. Activity should never be framed as punishment, e.g., "Turn off the video games and go out and run two miles, because you are too fat." Instead, an activity should be viewed as an extension of what is meaningful to the family, for example, like doing chores, completing homework, practicing the piano, walking the dog, helping out a family member or friend, or being a good listener.

The NFL had it right when naming their fitness and wellness initiative "Play 60," which now in its sixth year continues to gain momentum. Imagine if the NFL named it "Exercise 60?" What child (or average adult, for that matter) wants to exercise 60 minutes a day? To frame activity as play is to help turn the tide of inactivity among children that leads to inactivity in adulthood. While doctors and dieticians may prescribe exercise to address the agreed-upon key components of fitness (cardiovascular endurance, muscular strength, flexibility, and body composition), traditional exercise is proven to be much less effective than creating opportunities for play.

The best exercise for a particular child, despite any expert opinions to the contrary, is usually the activity that the child enjoys and is able to participate in safely. Prescribing the best exercise does little to benefit the child if they do not have the means to participate, do not like the activity, or cannot afford the time or dollars required to participate. The best exercise is also often one that the child determines is respected and valued by their family, culture, community, and themselves.

One of my friends had a son who loved to wrestle. He was not great at it, and the parents hated attending the unending weekend tournaments on high school bleachers. The teenager, however, was passionate about the sport, even during a stretch when he lost almost every single match. In reality, a self-selected physical activity may elicit a greater level of adherence than a physical activity prescribed by a parent, healthcare provider, or someone else.

BEYOND PERFECTION

Parenting is a tough job. In reality, parenting children is becoming even harder, given the reality of living in a culture that is obsessed with weight and is often governed by appearance fixations that wear down a child's sense of self. After decades of hearing the frustrations expressed by kids, I can sum up what I think they would say to their parents in their most honest moments:
- They want their parents to know how hard they try.
- They want them to know that pressuring (bribes, reminders, reprimand, lecture and punishment) weight loss only makes things worse.
- They want them to know that they often feel they have failed.
- They want them to know how much it hurts to know that they are a disappointment to their parents.
- They want them to know that they deeply feel shame and guilt.

- They want to live up to their expectations.
- They want to make things better but just don't know how.
- They want to ask for help, but feel embarrassed and fearful to do so.
- They worry that there must be something wrong with them, because of the fact that they can't do this right.

In their honest moments our children would also tell us that they long for the foods that are restricted and believe that eating just might help ameliorate their pain. They would tell us how humiliating it feels to go to the doctor and how shopping for clothes, something that could be fun, only makes them feel worse. They would say that they feel un-liked, often lonely, and that they fear they will forever be burdened by weight. At times, they may even say that they want to just give up on living.

I have a friend with four children, three of whom are teenagers, who has two children who are overweight. Both were bullied in middle school. Both lost elementary-school friends, once puberty hit. The parents struggled to know what to do to encourage them to engage in sound eating and exercise habits. They wondered what to say when noticing one of their children was drinking too much high sugar soda or seemingly taking too many snacks. The father, especially, mentioned how difficult it was to know what to say or not say regarding his daughter's eating habits observed in the middle of dinner. Should he pester her about eating or working out?

He would currently claim that while they have made their mistakes, over time, they learned to manage many pieces of this puzzle well. That particular daughter is now 15. On her own, she asks her parents to drive her to a sports facility to work out after dinner three times a week. Each day for school, she makes a lunch that always includes fruits and vegetables. Has she lost every possible pound of excess weight? No. But she now owns the process. She makes her choices. She is in charge.

Their son, 13, just started to see his weight stabilize after four years of dramatic increases. Recently, the son announced that he had "dropped five pounds." The boy told his dad, not only am I eating less these days, but I'm also not as hungry. The father said he was tempted to give his son a fist bump for the weight loss, but instead said, "You sound like you are proud of yourself! It also sounds like things are feeling easier. Good for you!" He tried courageously to focus on the behavior, as opposed to on the number or the weight loss per se.

While both children are making progress with their weight, the really great success is that they are doing it on their own. Once they let go of the concept of attaining perfection, the journey of parenting becomes more manageable, and the progress more sustainable. Even more importantly, the children involved will have a shot at achieving a more satisfying life.

Importantly, can parents work toward focusing on the whole person, seeing beyond the numbers, minimizing the level of importance assigned to their children's appearance, and recognizing and cultivating the internal qualities that are the more valued and essential components of their children's character and well-being?

Parenting is not without error for anyone. It is not an easy road, and there are no quick fixes.

8

Grading on a Scale

When the siren wailed, the first-grade class had 20 minutes to reach the top of the hill. It was the school's monthly tsunami evacuation drill. Every first-grader dashed up the steep incline. Except Jackson. He trudged up the hill. His weight beleaguered his breathing. As the gap widened between the boy and his peers, Jackson's teachers worried he might collapse. A quarter of the way up, Jackson stopped—his face beet-red—and refused to take another step.

"If it were an actual evacuation," a teacher wondered, "what would we have done?" The teachers' collective brawn couldn't drag the 165-pound first-grader to safety. One teacher of the Oregon coast elementary school recalls school officials telling her, "In the event of a real evacuation, such children would have to be left behind."

As America's educational system is singularly focused on leaving no child behind academically, it is leaving behind over 12 million obese children. Some individuals argue, in fact, that the passage of "No Child Left Behind" may be one of the many reasons that weight is a problem for one in three American children. As schools stare at potential penalties for not measuring up in reading, writing, and math, many schools have reduced or eliminated physical education and recess. Patricia Anderson and Kristin Butcher studied the factors contributing to childhood obesity, concluding that the academic system is partially to blame. "Children's health is not among the outcomes for which schools are held accountable" they wrote. "Schools facing accountability pressure may well make decisions designed to increase test scores that have unintended negative consequences for children's weight."

To stop the obesity epidemic requires a hard look at our educational system and its contribution to the problem. Our educators can play a significant role in improving the health of our children - and thus an entire generation, as they become adults.

THE POWER OF RECESS

Physical activity fuels brain power, as it improves the flow of blood and oxygen to the brain, as well as mood-improving chemicals. Yet since the passage of "No Child Left Behind" in 2001, 44 percent of school administrators report significant cuts in physical education (PE) and recess. The best evidence for not scaling back recess and PE might be a visit to a classroom of squirmy 4th graders denied activity throughout the day. Despite the sweeping evidence of the benefits of physical activity—all of which contribute to learning—school systems continue to trim or cut physical education and recess. While the National Association for Sports and Physical Education (NASPE) recommends that schools provide 150 minutes of instructional physical education for elementary school children each week, and 225 minutes for middle- and high-school students per week for the entire school year, only six states require physical education in every grade, K-12, according to the 2012 Shape of the Nation report. Furthermore, of these states, it isn't mandated every day. Only 2 percent require daily PE for all grades, all years in school. Loopholes also exist for students to opt out of PE altogether.

Recess may be kids' favorite subject, but they're not getting much of it. The NASPE recommends that children receive 20 minutes of recess a day, but only 59 percent of districts require schools to provide recess. In fact, students at the highest risk for obesity attend schools that are less likely to offer recess. In 2001, when No Child Left Behind was instituted, America's students enjoyed on average 37 minutes a day of recess; in 2008, the average dropped to 24 to 27 minutes.

America might benefit from emulating Finland, a nation that provides its students with 75 minutes of recess a day—15-minute breaks after each lesson. Finland ranks academically higher than the U.S. What makes recess so important? It's where students reach, on average, 40 percent of their total daily activity. Not only does it affect their weight, it apparently helps improve classroom attentiveness and behavior.

In the United States, some school officials punish students by taking away recess. If the homework isn't done, for instance, recess is denied, the very activity that could help refocus the child.

One result of decreased school activity, of course, is that children today are less physically fit than children of their parents' generation. At the 2013 American Heart Association's national meeting, research was presented that showed endurance among children dropped on average 6 percent each decade between 1970 and 2000. Children ran slower and shorter distances than children from their parents' generation. The unfortunate conclusion is that today's children are unhealthier than yesterday's children, and will eventually become tomorrow's unhealthier adults.

It's the refrain of our nation's Let's Move campaign: our children aren't moving enough. Only 25 percent of U.S. youth (ages 12 to15) participate in the recommended 60 minutes or more of moderate to vigorous activity every day. Just 13 percent of children walk or bike to school, because of perceived physical risk due to unsafe (or non-existent) walking routes. For some children, walking to school is indeed risky—gang-related violence, no sidewalks on busy streets, perilous neighborhood, etc.

For other students, their parents simply prefer the quick drop-off a few minutes before the bell. The onus is placed on the parent and child to clock in their 60 minutes after school. Few do. After-school hours are crammed with homework and screen time (mostly screen time), which obviate physical activity.

When asked, "How does the absence of physical activity at your school impact your child?" one parent of a Chicago Public School student said, "It is impossible for me to provide enough exercise time for my 3rd grader anymore. By the time we get home, do homework, have dinner, practice his musical instrument, it is time for bed. It used to be we had time [for him] to play at the park … time to be a kid." Compounding the problem is the fact that students aren't picking up the bat, putting on their shin guards, or hitting the mats outside of school hours. By age 13, 70 percent of youth who participate in organized sports drop out. As a result, children are more sedentary than ever.

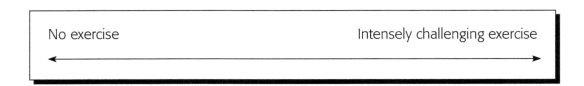

No exercise   Intensely challenging exercise

SCHOOL FOOD—THE GOOD AND THE BAD

One response to our education system's complicity in the childhood obesity epidemic is to increase the minutes of daily activity. Arguably, that's a good start.

As important as activity is, though, so is nutrition. In fact, some schools are reducing the caloric and fat content of their school menus, adding whole grains and fresh produce. That's the good news.

Children eat between one-third and one-half of their daily calories at school. With the passage of the Healthy Hunger-Free Kids Act in 2010, lunches are less like fast food and more like the government's "My Plate" recommendations. Not only are participating schools provided resources to purchase produce from local gardens and farms, they also are eligible for Federal reimbursement if they meet the new caloric and nutritional standards set by the USDA. A half-cup of fruits or vegetables and servings of at least two other foods, like a protein and a grain, must make their way onto a student's tray in order for schools to be funded.

To make the foods more palatable, a competition sponsored by the USDA challenged the public to develop flavorful, yet healthy, recipes for the school cafeteria. Even the tastiest recipes, however, don't tend to woo the taste buds of a teen's finely developed fast-food palate. As a result, school cafeteria staff are learning the complexity of providing healthy meals that won't go from tray to the trash.

After a year of trading in tater-tots and corn-dogs for pepper-laden chicken salad, however, schools are complaining that they're losing money, despite the reimbursement. Though change takes time, many schools are throwing caloric caution to the wind and again are dishing up fish sticks and fries.

Healthy school lunches will do little to contribute to a child's health, if schools don't limit competitive foods. Students unimpressed with (and unsatisfied by) the salad bar are tempted by the snacks displayed in vending machines. Such snacks, typically high in sugar, fat, coloring, and preservatives, threaten the health of our children. Research indicates that about 40 percent of all students buy and eat one or more snacks at school, and 68 percent buy and consume at least one sugary drink.

In 2014, one study revealed that 84 percent of high schools had contracts with beverage companies, like Coke and Pepsi. Some states are demanding their vending machines and school stores jettison the junk and replace it with options that have fewer empty calories, e.g., fruit candies for fruit cups, a chocolate bar for a granola bar, a soda for no-calorie flavored water. It's still expensive, but at least it's not pure fat and sugar.

Paying attention to the school's vending machines means paying attention to the health of the student body. One landmark study reported that students from states that enforced regulation of competitive foods gained less weight than individuals who attended school in states that didn't enforce laws. While educators may have good intentions of restocking their vending machines with healthier options, they often unwittingly fill them with more junk (e.g., fruit juice, instead of cola; fruit snacks, instead of Skittles). Frequently, the replacements have the same amount of empty calories as that which they replaced. Although there's been some progress, there's still a long way to go.

Even if every state cleaned up their vending machines and snack bars, the weekly class celebration has become practically a new sport that no one is winning. Some parents read the memo, strictly forbidding all items with fat and refined sugar. As a consequence, the compliant parents pack sliced peppers and rice cakes, while the afterschool gang gathers in the home that houses the cookies and potato chips. Other kids may unknowingly arrive with the preferred cookies or cupcakes to share. Their smiles quickly turn to shame and embarrassment. As they see the shaking heads of disapproval, they pack up their treats to take them back home.

FOCUS ON NUMBERS

The American education system is divided into two camps: winning schools in which no child is left behind, and losing schools in which too many children are. The national gold medal schools that top the yearly *U.S. News and World Report* report on the best high schools are the winners of the winners, quite simply because they produce more winners: National Merit Scholars, students who graduate with 5.0 GPAs, and the not-community-college-bound. In these schools, numbers, grades, and rankings measure success and, more importantly, human worth.

Arguably, the focus of educators on numbers is why nearly 20 states are turning to school-based BMI reporting to tackle childhood obesity. A number represents the tangible, the measurable, a known entity, or a mutually understood and agreed-upon target. Measured by points, obesity feels quantifiable and, therefore, solvable. As such, it's merely a matter of fixing a number. BMI screening is built upon the assumption that parents don't fully grasp that their child is overweight and will likely become an overweight adult. If more parents only knew that their child was obese or trending toward being obese, then, the thinking goes, motivation would kick in to correct the problem.

While advocates of school-based BMI screening point to research indicating that parents underestimate their child's weight, often the numbers are not accurately represented. For instance, a study of 742 mothers of adolescents found that 35 percent underestimated their child's weight status, and five percent overestimated it. In other words, a majority of parents accurately assessed their child's weight.

Parents who are notified of a problem with their child's weight often already know their child struggles with weight. Many parents have fought the weight battle with their children only to see their kid increase in weight, their self-esteem plummet, and/or their child slip into an eating disorder. Will a BMI letter help them guide their child on a path to health? BMI screenings may create more problems than they solve. Just as a failing school's cumulative standardized test scores aren't necessarily reflective of its quality, hardworking students, and dedicated teachers, a BMI chart does not reflect a child's entire health picture. BMI screenings fail to account for cultural beliefs and values about weight. For instance, some cultures are more accepting of extra weight and less likely to perceive themselves as being overweight. In addition, they tend to demonstrate a greater level of body satisfaction.

To alert minority parents that their child is overweight or obese is to raise concern that many cultures may not perceive as concerning. BMI notifications sent home with recommendations about healthful living are often ineffectual, when environmental and cultural barriers, including beliefs and values, stand in the way.

School-based BMI screenings also don't entirely account for a child's eating and exercise patterns, psycho-behavioral patterns, and family and health history, as well as biological factors (which are often elements that are taken into consideration by a family physician). Schools hold only one piece of the puzzle.

A "Good Morning America" news story pointed to this exact problem. In this feature, Ali, an 11-year-old girl from Florida, was sent home with a "fat letter," after a BMI screening at her school. The letter informed her parents that Ali's BMI was concerning. If it was not addressed, she risked being overweight the rest of her life. Ali, however, is not overweight. A volleyball player who snacks on carrots and peppers, Ali could be a poster child for the Let's Move campaign.

Ali was hurt, her parents furious. "To give a kid a letter telling them that the rest of their life they may be overweight or they may be obese because of a measurement you took one day," said Ali's mother, "it's just not fair." As in many cases, the BMI measurement belied the actual health of the child.

If a child has real health concerns related to weight, a BMI screening does not guarantee a solution. Research shows that while "most parents" don't oppose BMI screening (if done in a confidential manner), they generally don't follow-up with a medical-care provider after receiving their child's screening results. Physicians in Arkansas where BMI screening is required confirm this point. Many parents, in fact, place their child on a diet, without consulting a doctor or dietician. It could be the first diet of many to follow, in which restrictions feed the craving for the forbidden. For some individuals, BMI screening can trigger a lifetime of weight cycling.

School-based BMI screenings also rouse dread and insecurity among students who already fret endlessly about how they are perceived by peers. One student reported that as she stood in line for her weight measurement, her teacher's eyes widened when her heavier friend's weight was measured. Curious students hovered around the scale, as the student cowered in shame. When "Good Morning America" interviewed a panel of teens about BMI screenings, one 13-year-old teen girl, Lucy, said, "I'm insecure because I'm taller than a lot of girls in my school. Furthermore, I'm also bigger than a lot of them. I'm not incredibly skinny." It's the "not-incredibly-skinny" girls—the ones who wish they knew how to drop 15 pounds—who fall in the danger zone. To be sent home with a "fat letter" is to be a target for fat jokes or the recipient of sideways glances and snickering. It can also cause a girl to cry herself to sleep; to feel anxious about going to gym class; and to undertake extreme or risky dieting.

One option is to send home letters confidentially. In reality, however, students will still compare their scores, just like they do their mile-run times in gym class or math-placement test scores. This situation leads to, "Did you hear that Jake had a BMI of 40?" Suddenly, kids have a new taxonomy for good (BMI $\leq$ 24) and bad (BMI $>$ 24). For students already worried about their weight, comparison invites feelings of self-hatred and increased anxiety. This scenario, in turn, can lead to crashing self-esteem, eating disorders, and even, in the extreme, suicide.

While BMI measurement can be a helpful tool for scientists and epidemiologists to monitor trends in a population, it does not provide useful information about body composition, such as percentages of bone, muscle, and fat. Furthermore, BMI testing and reporting does not provide guidance for parents or students for understanding and managing health and eating constructively thereafter. BMI testing and reporting is neither a valid nor a reliable tool for helping students become healthy children or adults.

FAT ATTITUDES IN THE CLASSROOM

While not intended, "fat letters" are an extension of the weight discrimination already occurring in schools. Two decades ago, when the "Just Say No" campaign was wrapping up its war against adolescent drug abuse, the National Education Association (NEA) was tuning into the rumblings of another problem facing America's youth. An NEA executive committee, focused on fostering healthy learning environments, compiled a report highlighting the anti-fat attitudes and behaviors seething in America's schools. In "The Report on Size Discrimination," the committee wrote:

> For fat students, the school experience is one of ongoing prejudice, unnoticed discrimination, and almost constant harassment. From nursery school through college, fat students experience ostracism, discouragement, and sometimes violence. Often ridiculed by their peers and discouraged by even well-meaning education employees,

fat students develop low self-esteem and have limited horizons. They are deprived of places on honor rolls, sports teams, and cheerleading squads and are denied letters of recommendation."

The findings of the report are as real today as they were 20 years ago. As more kids are obese, the amount of weight discrimination grows.

The fat-is-bad, fat-is-ugly, fat-is-lazy stereotypes adopted by children during their preschool years often manifests as discrimination during their grade-school and adolescent years. A 2015 study found that 6 out of 10 overweight youth experience weight-based victimization at school, mainly in the form of teasing or exclusion. Of the perpetrators, 92 percent were peers, 70 percent were friends, 42 percent were physical education teachers/coaches, and 27 percent were teachers.

A person does not have to be the victim to recognize that the victimization is occurring. Furthermore, an individual does not need to be overweight to be teased about their weight. In a survey of high-school students, 92 percent reported incidents of overweight youth being ridiculed. "Fatso" (or some variation thereof) is as common to the youth dialect as "dude." In school hallways, gym class, math class, and cafeterias, overweight students are caught in the anti-fat crossfire.

The more disheartening story, though, is not only the attitudes of students. It's also the overt weight bias on display by teachers themselves. A student tells the story of being assigned one of two classroom desks that were smaller than the rest of the classroom desks. When he couldn't fit into the desk, his knees scraping the base of the metal top, he asked to be placed in a different seat. Rather than quietly accommodate the student, the teacher demanded he sit in it again to prove his point. After struggling to get back in the seat, the teacher responded, "Wow. You are fat!" and moved him to the front of the classroom to a table. She said, "I'm going to name this the obese table for kids who can't seem to control their fat."

This story is a patently egregious anecdote. Worse, perhaps, is the subtle weight discrimination that sits just beneath the surface of the attitudes and behaviors of some of today's educators. Most often, if a teacher discriminates against a child who is obese, it's unintentional, as well as subtle. In reality, many teachers don't realize that they are expressing biases. Like doctors, parents, and peers, teachers are subject to the prevailing views of the culture. As such, they're drunk on the thin ideal, which likely has surrounded them for a lifetime.

Teachers' negative stereotypes of obese students—such as, they are more emotional, less tidy, less likely to succeed at work—are an offshoot of fat hatred. Recently, a University of New Mexico psychology instructor took some heat after tweeting that doctoral candidates who "don't have the willpower to stop eating carbs won't have the willpower to do a dissertation." Often, such stereotypes are more strongly expressed by physical education instructors who possess strong ideological beliefs about physical fitness.

As might be imagined, implicit (and explicit) biases can derail a student's educational experience. Heavier elementary children, for instance, miss more school than their normal-weight classmates. Adolescents who have experienced weight discrimination report that they struggle to perform academically. Furthermore, obese adolescent girls are less likely than their non-obese peers to attend college.

Ironically, the very strategies schools employ to tackle obesity often lead to increased discrimination. At Prospect High School in the Chicago suburb of Mt. Prospect, administrators created a physical education program, wherein students were divided into a "lower" or "higher" class, depending on their physical fitness levels. Thin students labeled it "fat gym"—because as one Prospect student said, "It was like a division of the fat kids and the thin kids."

Its name is only one of the reasons this program is discriminatory. Students placed in the "lower fat" gym class reportedly get to pick activities and sports they want to pursue. Students who are placed in the "higher fat" class are forced into mandatory cardio programs three days a week. Again, the traditional paradigm emerges: thin is rewarded, fat is punished.

Weight-related bias does not just hurt those individuals who are targets. Everyone is a victim of such bias. As such, everyone loses. Families observe the hurt. Friends see the hurt. Educators see the disruption in relationships, classroom mood, and motivation to learn. Judgment and bias do not just injure their victims. They hurt all who witness such actions, a group that includes themselves. In fact, attempting to feel "better than" by making others feel "less than" is an endless and defeating path.

As a nation, we need to recognize, as the NEA did 20 years ago, that perhaps the first place to start is addressing the weight biases that exist within our educational system and are crippling our children's sense of worth. Educators can begin by reflecting on their own biases, while also modeling and reinforcing non-discriminatory attitudes: Do they falsely believe that overweight students are lazy, unlikeable, disorganized, and thus less likely to succeed? Do they inappropriately favor students who aren't overweight?

Unfortunately, all humans are subject to bias of some kind. This scenario is never an easy reality to admit. Few educators want to admit that they are biased or treat students differently. It's uncomfortable for them to absorb the situation fully. The data, however, shows otherwise: teacher perception affects grades. It's the kind of subtle bias that must be admitted by teachers, before it can be addressed.

HOW CHANGE BEGINS

Exercise, nutrition, less focus on metrics, and addressing weight bias—all need to be components of strategies that educators take into consideration as they address the childhood obesity epidemic. *It's not simply one thing. It's a million things. A million little fixes in every sphere of the culture.* Educators must look beyond the numbers and create an environment that sets up students for success in the present, as well as a lifetime of health in the future. As such, eating decisions today create patterns that affect students for a lifetime. More importantly, decisions that can impact our children's well-being for generations to come are extremely important and must be undertaken with the utmost forethought.

It's not simply tactics, however, but thinking about the larger picture. For example, what is the role of exercise in the life of our students? Students age 9 to 18 who are physically active are more likely to be physically active adults. Recess allows students to explore, relate to others, and, ultimately, become fully human, i.e., complete.

An argument is often advanced for more competitive sports programs, but ones that don't demand specialization and groom super-stardom at an early age. In fact, support exists for reducing exposure to competitive sports at such early ages. Competition creates winners and losers; it results in a score; it tells children that they are good or bad, successful or not. A number of children aren't ready for that. Rather than cutting the sports budget, the education system would do better to invest in more fields, gyms, and courts—so every child has a place to participate if they are interested and have fun doing so.

"Girls on the Run" is one such after-school activity that takes competition out of the equation. The program was developed to help girls, through running, to "activate [their] limitless potential." One mother, who was concerned about her pre-teen daughter's activity level, was immediately drawn to the program. Her daughter, she said, wasn't athletic by typical standards. They had signed her up for soccer, but she never felt "good enough." Her confidence only waned.

"Girls on the Run" changed things. "There is no weight requirement. Girls do not need a perfect body. They don't need to be coordinated," says the mother. The program includes healthy food and healthy body discussion. The program combats the "You've got to be skinny to be important" message that crushes the spirit of our nation's children. After successfully completing her first 5K, her daughter continued running throughout the summer (and encouraged her mom to start running, too!). Activity, she realized, was empowering—even fun.

Schools can also create more opportunities for activity breaks during classroom time. These activities can range from the more traditional (10 minutes of stretching or chair aerobics prior to a class session) to the more playful and creative (play an age-appropriate song, perhaps related to a component of the curriculum, and allow students to dance; or have students act out a story, rather than just listen to a story).

Activity and learning aren't mutually exclusive. In fact, activity can be used to teach math, science, social studies, and character development. One teacher reported that gardening with her 4th graders promoted learning and health on multiple levels. Not only did it help them understand basic components of biology, it also taught a sense of personal responsibility, through the regular activity of weeding and watering, as well as an appreciation of nutrition. Of the experience, she stated that the students "learned to take ownership of the food they put into bodies and gained an understanding of how those foods could help them feel strong and healthy. Its focus on nutrition and health was a refreshing shift from all the talk about avoiding obesity."

FOOD IN THE DAY OF A STUDENT

What is the purpose of eating in the life of a student? What will optimize learning? Food is not a stand-alone function, like seventh-period Calculus. Food is what the body needs to function 24 hours a day. In fact, having lunch at brunch time is common at many overcrowded schools. From pre-K through high school, students are eating lunch as early as 9:30 in the morning. Often, students are forced to eat at inconvenient times in order to accommodate their schedules.

At a minimum, students should always have access to water and snacks throughout the day and during athletic practice. Improved frequency of eating, as well as availability of healthy food and drink options, rather than eating regulated by rules and restrictions, helps children to be able to respond mindfully and responsibly to their hunger. Being mindful is paying attention to their own body and its needs.

Educators must persist in the hard work of supplying healthy lunch and snack options, even when opposition mounts. Schools facing resistance to changing school menus must keep in mind that the bigger the change, the harder it is to be successful. Just as a child doesn't go from riding a tricycle to doing tricks on a BMX, a child doesn't go from eating processed, preservative-laden, frozen pizza to overnight consuming a well-balanced meal without adjustment or resistance.

To get from A to Z may require small, gradual steps in between. The trick is to gradually replace unhealthy options with healthier alternatives: whole grains, more fresh fruits and vegetables, less processed food, and lower-fat options. It is important to remember that humans often have difficulty unlearning entrenched patterns and relearning new ones, food-related or not.

It will be beneficial for schools and school districts to rethink the role of food in their institution, to allow ample time for eating. Kelly Brownell argues in *Food Fight* that our fast-food culture has resulted in "toxic food environments," a factor that has largely changed our culture's values toward eating. Before fast food fueled Americans, we sat around the table for meals and used flatware that didn't break and dishes that just might. Families slowed down their days enough to enjoy their food, as well as to engage in conversation. Now, we eat with our hands from Styrofoam plates and drink from straws, while standing up, driving in cars, or working at a desk. In fact many students may know more about the content of fast foods than family recipes. Today, schools may complicit in perpetuating a toxic food environment, rushing students through meals and permitting sales of cheaper, competitive processed foods.

Crowded schools and crowded schedules leave little time for lunch. Some students complain that it takes too long to eat. Applesauce slides down quickly, but eating an apple takes time. Diane Pratt-Heavner, spokeswoman for the School Nutrition Association, a national advocacy organization, says, "If we want our students to eat more salads, fruits, and vegetables, we need to give them more time to consume them."

Students may wait in line first for a ticket to eat food and then in another line for the food itself. They may also have to wait to find an available seat or wait for one to be vacated. In fact, a number of students don't have a full 30 minutes to eat. Students who don't have time to eat often won't eat anything.

As a result, students suffer the consequences of hunger, like distraction, stomach aches, and behavioral problems. Students also miss vitally important time to talk, relax, connect with friends, and exchange ideas. Furthermore if they're hungry, they may overeat at the convenience store across the street after school. Students race to receive food, eat the food, and then race to the next class.

This scenario is not mindful eating. Mindfulness is critical in helping students listen to their body and sustain healthy eating practices. While slowing down meals at school is countercultural, it is vital in allowing students time to refuel, refresh, and connect with their peers.

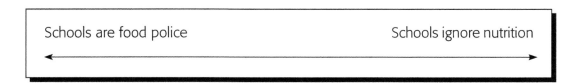

Schools are food police   Schools ignore nutrition

New strategies may facilitate new approaches. When it comes to classroom celebrations, for pre-K and elementary educators in particular, it has become complicated. In previous generations, before store-bought cupcakes, doughnuts, and cookies were par-for-the-course for class parties, parents would make homemade desserts for celebrations. The situation has changed.

At the present time, "healthy" foods are encouraged or, in some cases, required. Seems like a useful strategy, but who determines how "healthy" is defined? What if some children are allergic to "healthy"? Must teachers read the label on every snack that enters the classroom to review the contents of the food item? Are children needing to get in line before entering the lunch room to have their lunch bags searched for contraband? If high-sugar and high-fat foods are listed on the "forbidden food" list, do they become the most preferred binge food? Are teachers being asked to become the food police? Can parents really add another morning debate about food and nutritional content, before the child leaves for school each day?

There are solutions, but they will likely stem from much thoughtful collaboration among teachers, parents, healthcare providers, school policymakers and community health experts. Change will not be instantaneous. Change must be gradual. It is also important to remember that one rule will not work for all students. In the meantime, it may be helpful to be creative. Celebrations can be celebratory without food. New traditions and practices can be adopted to celebrate accomplishments, birthdays, and culminating activities, for example, a note, a tradition, applause, a goodbye book of collected messages from all students in the class, walking the hall of fame, adding to a gratefulness list for friendship or learning, verbally acknowledging a success, a name posted on the "star of the day" sign, etc.

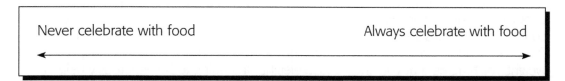

The more educators can, they should resist the temptation to reward students with candy or other food, or punish children by taking away recess or other activities. Although such a strategy may work, as a rule, it is typically a temporary and only a very short-term solution. Unfortunately, using food and exercise this way reduces more internal focus and awareness. It may also diminish more intrinsic interest in exercise and healthy eating. Rewarding or punishing students with food strengthens the relationship between food and behavior. This situation is potentially a powerful relationship that may be detrimental over time.

A BIAS-FREE ZONE

Another more strategic issue is the message that the school sends to students through the curriculum. Does the curriculum advance the values the school wants to communicate to students about the role of food in their life, physical activity, nutrition, and the cultural biases about weight? Is there a way to learn the principles of health in a way that doesn't communicate that fat is bad, thin is good, and everyone who is not perceived as thin is unhealthy?

While students certainly need more information about health, it can be delivered in a manner that reframes the current cultural issues about health in nuanced and fresh ways. Students need a size-neutral curriculum that reflects our cultural and bodily diversity. Stereotypes will always exist. Accordingly, a number of books may need to be rewritten to minimize these stereotypes. Do the images all support the cultural bias of the thin ideal? Throughout the school environment, are diverse body types respected?

Furthermore, school districts should be urged to employ non-discriminatory grading practices. Research shows that grading improves when the teacher connects the person with the test. Ergo, appearance affects grades. This factor correlates with the research of doctors who perceive patients as lazy, based on their weight. A recent study of musicians revealed that the highest score from the judges could be predicted, based on the appearance of the musician (without hearing the music!).

The relevance of the appearance factor is illustrated by the story of a teacher, who moonlights as a personal fitness trainer. This teacher recently became aware of how her own weight bias made its way into her classroom. She remembers how one sixth-grade student, in passing, made a comment about having "love handles." Teachers love to help their students, and they love to teach. This teacher wanted to help this student.

The teacher told the student that she "was available to help her work on feeling better about her body" if she wanted. The teacher then realized her mistake. Her comment could easily be translated by the student as something less-than-supportive, for example, "Yes, love handles are bad and should be corrected." "I know how to help you lose weight," or "I agree that you should lose weight." Intending to be generously helpful, the comments could have been perceived as additional criticism. In fact, students may have already felt they have "tried," and they have "failed." Hearing more about "solutions" and the need for change may deepen their sense of failure.

How do teachers confront their own biases about weight? It's not easy. First, they need to have an enhanced level of awareness of pervasive cultural weight bias. Self-awareness can help, but it is not always a simple process. Many educators may want to fix their overweight students, without recognizing the complexity of their struggle or the messages that the teachers unintentionally send, on occasion. Offering to help "fix the problem" highlights the fact that having "love handles" is a "problem" that can and should be changed.

Our culture has taught us all to respond this way. Teachers who instinctively jump in to help are doing what they love to do: helping kids. Not all fixes, however, can make this situation better. In fact, some solutions might make things worse. Changing these instinctive responses might mean delaying the response, considering the short- and longer-term options, listening more, avoiding the offer of an immediate solution, and remaining compassionate.

Identifying the strengths in our children can be helpful in many situations. For example, "I noticed how you showed leadership in my class today." And, "I am seeing excellent cooperation right now." In the landmark study on teacher's beliefs about obese students, leading researcher Dianne Neumark-Sztainer says, "Since school staff have ongoing contact with many youth, they are in a unique position … to help overweight students feel better about themselves in a thin-oriented society."

Helping kids feel better about their bodies will benefit more than just their attitudes and beliefs about weight and shape. It will also help them have more confidence to successfully learn, to have relationships, and to pursue educational opportunities that are satisfying. In fact, a more positive self-perception will permit more positive living in general.

One morning, an elementary school teacher walked into the bathroom and heard rustling from one of the stalls. When the girl came out, the teacher saw her fisting a bag of potato chips. Heavier than the rest of her peers, the girl said she was eating, because she was hungry. Her mom had placed her on a diet. Tears ran down her face as she said, "But, I am starving. My lunch isn't enough!" More confessions followed, including the shame she felt for being "fat" and how other students ridiculed her because of her size.

After speaking with her mother, the teacher stocked the cupboards and classroom refrigerator with fruits, vegetables, and healthy snacks. She also allowed more frequent snack time, if the students were hungry. She declared a moratorium on reference to size and shape in her classroom. She made classroom rules about "fat talk," commenting on what anyone eats and other discriminatory language.

The teacher also began incorporating lessons about embracing individual differences and avoiding an overemphasis on either fat or thin. She shared the benefits and burdens of different body types: "Being tall is awesome, when you need to reach something, but a bummer when you want to be comfortable in airplane seating. Shorter people can fit into small spaces and easily scramble to retrieve the pencil that rolls under the desk, but it might be harder for them to navigate their way through a crowd. Muscular bodies can be more resilient, when they fall, but it might be hard to find clothes that fit comfortably."

This teacher recommitted herself to establishing a more size-friendly environment in her classroom. She thought more about the related language used by students and herself. She reconsidered moments of differential attention based on size, shape, or weight. She became more mindful of images used in reading materials, video, and printed material, as well as the implicit and explicit messages they convey. She also looked for new learning resources that were less weight-biased.

Twenty years ago, when our daughter was five-years old, we were seated at a long and crowded table of 18 friends and family for a holiday dinner. Conversation was interesting and lively. A quiet moment occurred as salt and pepper were passed among the guests. At that point, our daughter loudly announced, "Uncle George, you are fat!" In reality, Uncle George was a large, round and full-figured, successful stockbroker, who loved to play Santa, because he so naturally looked the part.

The moment quickly became even more quiet. Searching for something to say, I offered, "Yes. Uncle George is fat, and you are short. You have long hair, Uncle Phillip is tall, Grandma has red hair, and your father has big muscles." Isn't it nice that we are all different because if we all looked the same, I couldn't see which person was you at this table." As such, fat is perceived as "bad," simply because our culture has defined it as such.

The awareness and changes made by teachers are part of a larger and important whole. As a nation, we can do better. Educators and the education system can do better. We can arrive at a place where weight, shape, and size are not the only indicators of a person's worth or potential. We can provide a safe environment, in which students are prepared for a lifetime of success physically, emotionally, mentally, and behaviorally. We can help our children learn how to embrace who they uniquely are, to accept the body they have, and to define success in a way that works for them.

These efforts will take time. These efforts will meet resistance. These efforts won't be perfect. To do nothing, however, is to leave behind a generation of children struggling to live as content, confident, and successful humans.

9

The Exercise Culture in America

Americans spend more than 3.1 trillion dollars annually for healthcare. Over 70 percent of this figure is for care from preventable chronic disease. This meteoric figure means that $9,695 is dispensed yearly for every man, woman, and child in the United States for healthcare, or 26 cents of every single dollar spent in America is allocated for healthcare.

Attempts to identify the factors that contribute to poor health have produced an array of probable reasons for poor health, including unhealthy eating habits, a sedentary lifestyle, stress, smoking, etc. Studies have looked for factors that may reduce the number and severity of the medical problems affecting the public. As such, these efforts have provided considerable evidence that exercise has substantial medicinal benefit for individuals of all ages.

Two of the most widely publicized investigations of the relationship between exercise and disease were longitudinal studies. Each study included more than 10,000 individuals. In the first, conducted several years ago, in a renowned study of Harvard graduates, Ralph Paffenbarger, M.D., found that men who expended approximately 300 calories a day—the equivalent of walking briskly for 45 minutes—reduced their death rates from all causes by an extraordinary 28 percent.

In the second, a more recent study undertaken by Dr. Steven Blair, it was found that a relatively modest amount of exercise has a significant effect on the mortality rate of both men and women. The higher the fitness level, the lower the death rate (in an eight-year investigation of 13,344 individuals). In addition, Blair and his group discovered that even if a person is not initially fit and begins to participate in an exercise program – at any age, it is possible to decrease risk of premature death by up to 50 percent, compared to those individuals who don't exercise.

EXERCISE IS MEDICINE

An analysis of the extensive data yielded by both studies suggests one inescapable conclusion—exercise is "medicine." Dr. Blair concluded, for example, that *not exercising had the equivalent impact on a person's health of smoking one and one-half packs of cigarettes a day.* Unfortunately, fewer have recognized the extraordinary benefits of exercise in preventing and treating medical problems. Awareness of the premise that regular exercise can play a key role in reducing risk of medical problems and in decreasing the costs for healthcare is crucial. The value of exercising on a regular basis is irrefutable. Inexplicably, however, most Americans continue to live sedentary lives.

Much has been learned over the years about the role of exercise in promoting health. In that regard, the benefits of exercising are vast, varied, and irrefutable. For example, minutes of exercise are associated with longevity; exercise in senior years is associated with preserved cognitive function; exercise activity is associated with improved immune function and reduced risk of numerous illnesses and disease. In fact, the benefits have been repeatedly documented in study after study.

The data has been clear for some time. Remaining physically active throughout the day is vital to good health. Remaining physically active at least at a lower level of intensity reduces risk of disease and premature death.

UNDERSTANDING HEALTH RISK FACTORS

Knowing as much as possible about health and various risk factors can help inform and influence behavior choices. While health risk factors may indicate risk for certain diseases and medical conditions, self-care choices can minimize risk. Except for genetic factors (heredity, gender, and age), an individual has the opportunity to control most factors placing their health at risk. Much can be done to preserve and improve health.

❏ Uncontrollable Risk Factors:

The three health risk factors beyond control are age, sex, and family history. Age and sex interact, while family history stands alone. Understanding the specifics of these three factors can inform good health awareness, risk, and opportunity.

- *Age/sex:* Men over 45 years of age and women older than 55 (or post-menopausal women without estrogen replacement therapy) are at greater risk for debilitating disease than the general population.
- *Family history:* Unfortunately, no one has discovered a way to choose the right combination of DNA on a grand scale. Most everyone will inherit various genetic strengths and weaknesses. Individuals who have fathers or close male relatives who have had heart attacks or sudden death before age 55, or who have mothers or other close female relatives who've experienced the same condition(s) prior to 65 years of age, are at greater risk for serious disease than others.

Although there is nothing you can do about these three uncontrollable risk factors, recognizing them can help you better understand the importance of exerting control over the five factors that you CAN modify:

❏ Controllable Risk Factors:

Although a number of factors exist that are associated with disease and disability (and there are certainly others that will be discovered over the coming years), the most clearly understood of the controllable health risk factors are high blood pressure, high blood cholesterol, diabetes, cigarette smoking, and a sedentary lifestyle.

- *Sedentary lifestyle:* Long-range, medically-based studies of all-cause mortality point out the importance of not being sedentary. When the exercise habits of both men and women are examined over years of research, one of the most conclusive recommendations, relative to the relationship between physical activity and the level of premature death or disability is to "stay physically active over your lifetime."

Probably the most interesting finding of Steven Blair and his colleagues is that the most important predictor of living longer is not to be classified in the lowest fitness category. Although additional levels of fitness may increase how long a person lives, to a degree, their lifespan will not increase substantially. In other words, systematic exercise at relatively low levels will increase how long an individual lives almost as much as will more vigorous exercise. In that regard, an obese individual who exercises on a regular basis may be at a lower level of health risk than an inactive low-fat person who never exercises. The key point to be noted is that being physically active provides significant health benefits, regardless of a person's weight or "fat weight" condition.

THE OBESITY GENE

Genetics is known to powerfully influence the degree of obese condition. For example, carriers of mutations that exist in one gene, i.e., the FTO gene, which is present in nearly half of Europeans, are about 30 to 60 percent more likely to be fat. University of Maryland researchers decided to examine the FTO gene in the homogenous Amish community, since almost all of them are of European descent.

They found that, as with others of European descent, this gene did contribute to being overweight in the Amish community. The excess weight, however, was seen only in those individuals with low physical activity scores, such as women assigned to more in home and household responsibilities like cooking, cleaning, sewing, laundry, etc. The genetic phenotype did not present for those burning additional calories through several hours of moderately intensive physical exercise, such as farming, carpentry, etc.

At a very basic level the University of Maryland study confirms what has been suspected. Population-wide obesity is a modern phenomenon. We carry the same genes as our ancestors, but lifestyle change has fueled the obesity epidemic. Our bodies are changing in the face of the changing environment and lifestyle.

A PRESCRIPTION FOR HEALTH

If only people would exercise. Arguably, from a prescription standpoint, it involves adhering to a simple equation entailing *frequency* (the number of days per week with exercise), *intensity* (how hard to exercise to achieve results), *duration* (the number of minutes or hours engaged in exercise), and *mode* (the types of exercise used to optimize results). The *FIDM* equation should make it easier to reign in obesity in America.

This formula has been around for over 50 years, however. There is large scientific community support and widespread agreement that these are the fundamental components of safe and effective exercise. On the other hand, the resulting benefits of exercise for epidemic obesity are not clear. Even with access to the FIDM equation and its customary use for individual exercise prescription, the rates of obesity continue to escalate.

The majority of people at all socioeconomic levels are not engaged in activity as prescribed by FIDM. All factors considered, the FIDM structure seems to work well for competitive athletes. For the other 90 percent of the population who wish to decrease their risk of disease and live full and productive lives, however, a different model may be worthy of consideration.

As recently as 2016, the Centers for Disease Control reported that the number one cause of death among adults is cardiovascular disease (cancer of all types is still number five). In countless studies over the past 30 years, researchers have unequivocally demonstrated the beneficial relationship between fitness and the risk of developing chronic disease of all types. In fact, numerous researchers have demonstrated that exercise is good for health. More importantly, moving from a position of no physical activity to a moderate level of physical activity has been found to have a significant increase in the reduction of health-related risks of an individual.

While the FIDM model often recommends the highest possible fitness level, improved fitness at any level has significant health benefits. On the other hand, exercise regimens that are too intense can pose a higher risk of injury, less enjoyment, and greater recidivism. Lower intensity exercise, even for fewer minutes than recommended, can have a positive impact on a person's health.

HOW EXERCISE AFFECTS WEIGHT-RELATED HEALTH

The metabolic and psychological importance of exercise in weight control has been studied for many decades. For example, the results of a number of investigative efforts have documented the fact that exercise is associated with increased energy expenditure and increased metabolic rate during and after exercise. It is important to be aware of the fact that resting muscle cells utilize approximately three times more energy than fat cells. Exercise and physical activity conditions muscle mass, thereby preserving loss of muscle during periods of inactivity and hence maintaining basal metabolic rate. Longer-term exercise and a physically active lifestyle can preserve both muscle mass and increases in RMR (resting metabolic rate), even when fat mass and body mass are reduced.

Certainly, more needs to be learned about how the reactions in the body impact exercise and obesity. For example, it is hypothesized that regular exercise may have beneficial health effects on the hormones of the body that regulate energy balance. Adiponectin is secreted by fat cells and mediates metabolism of glucose and fatty acids. Higher levels of this hormone are associated with reduced risks of illnesses such as type 2 diabetes, atherosclerotic diseases, fatty liver disease, and metabolic syndrome. Exercise also increases SNS activity in people who have abnormally low tonic activity (i.e., physiological response) of the sympathetic nervous system. Furthermore, exercise can have positive psychological effects that help people adhere to dietary or exercise programs. In addition, exercise may improve mood and suppress appetite, as well as offset the effects of weight cycling.

COMMITMENT TO FITNESS: A LITTLE EXERCISE CAN GO A LONG WAY

Regular exercise can have a positive effect on both the duration and the quality of a person's life. In other words, exercise is associated with both improved longevity and improved functional capacity. Those individuals who exercise may live longer and live better. The impact of sound exercise on health and sense of well-being is substantial and well-documented. More importantly, exercise can substantially boost immune function and reduce the risk of contracting certain diseases and medical conditions, all of which are either caused by or worsened by being physically inactive.

In fact, small steps can collectively have a major impact on an individual's health. Although incremental acts, such as walking during a person's lunch hour, joining the local bowling league, or playing with their kids, etc., can seem inconsequential, they can make a noteworthy healthful difference. The value of a sound exercise program goes beyond improved longevity. Despite the plethora of documented information that exists concerning the benefits of exercise, participation across the United States remains very low. In fact, a recent government study estimates that nearly 80 percent of adult Americans don't get the recommended amount of exercise each week. Furthermore, only 34 percent of children in the United States exercise at least one hour per day, four days per week. Despite the plethora of documented information that exists concerning the benefits of exercise, participation across the United States remains very low. In fact, a recent government study estimates that nearly 80 percent of adult Americans don't get the recommended amount of exercise each week. Furthermore, only 34 percent of children in the United States exercise at least one hour per day, four days per week.

ATTITUDES AND PRACTICE IN EXERCISE AND PHYSICAL ACTIVITY

An exercise trainer worked two to three times per week with a 40-something male client for several years. When the client, who often traveled for business, was out of town, he scheduled workout sessions with trainers in other cities and states in order to help keep weight and eating frustrations in check. For many years, he felt he weighed more than he preferred to weigh. Over time, he had lost some weight, given his utilization of exercise trainers, having workouts locked into his schedule, engaging in psychotherapy to help deal with stress, making a concerted effort to learn about nutrition, and generally adhering to healthy decisions about food.

On one recent spring day, the trainer arrived and checked in briefly with him about how he was feeling. He then proposed the workout plan for the morning, given the client's interests. Upon hearing that the client had signed on for the upcoming summer volleyball league, he suggested an exercise plan for the day that would help the client prepare for summer beach volleyball. The trainer proposed targeting cardiac endurance, muscular endurance, flexibility, balance, and joint-risk reduction exercises, anticipating the uneven playing surface, the fast-paced activity, the heat, and the sun.

The client thought the plan sounded acceptable, discussed the details for few minutes with the trainer, and then got started. Several minutes later, the client offered the following observation, "You know," he said, "You are the only trainer I have ever had that does not talk to me about my weight. Thanks."

It is often the case that a person's weight is mentioned when that individual is seeing an exercise specialist. Weight can also be a common topic of discussion when calling on a physician, shopping for clothes, filling out insurance forms, and, even for some individuals, when purchasing plane tickets. At times, the discussion of weight may be lifesaving and pertinent. At other times, it can reduce someone to feeling like little more than a number on the scale.

Often, the discussion becomes a reminder of "not being good enough" in some way. Some trainers may venture into discussions about "recommended weights" and offer diet advice, provide protein shakes, or launch descriptions of their own personal weight-loss strategies. While well-intended, these practices may do more harm than good.

WHY AMERICANS MIGHT NOT LIKE TO ENGAGE IN EXERCISE OR PHYSICAL ACTIVITY

Not everyone loves exercise or physical activity. A number of reasons can account for having such attitude. Some individuals can recall being asked to do push-ups or run the track as punishment during physical education or as a member of an athletic team. Others remember being in physical education classes that had a limited array of activities, uninspiring instruction, poor facilities, or an environment in which they experience moments of embarrassment or shame in them that left lasting impressions.

Many of these individuals did not grow up in households where physical activity, for example, hanging out with friends, shooting hoops or throwing a ball, was enjoyed and modeled by parents or other family members. Some did not have access to safe parks, pools, or recreational facilities. A number of them currently view physical activity or exercise merely as a way "to burn calories," as opposed to a means to have some fun. When engaging in competitive sports, most adults found it challenging to continue their childhood sports interests into adulthood. In fact, trends for children in competitive sports indicate that many youth are leaving sport earlier than in previous generations. Furthermore, research suggests a variety of factors, such as stress, coach/athlete conflict, frustrations with time management, family finances, and parental pressures to excel, may also contribute to early dropout from sports.

FOCUSING ON THE NUMBERS

One 20-something client had worked for almost a year to improve her healthy eating, become more physically active, stop weighing herself obsessively, and think about her health in terms of her attitude and acceptable body curves. She had limited access to exercise options in her neighborhood, but eventually found the courage to try a health/ fitness club near her place of employment. She got creative about her haircut and putting her hair in a style that could survive a quick shower and facilitate a rapid return to the office after her lunch break.

On day one of her new health/fitness club membership, a trainer welcomed her, gave her a tour, and then began an anthropomorphic and fitness assessment, including weight, body composition, circumference measurements, and tests for flexibility, strength, and endurance. Her scores were posted on graphs, comparing her results with others normed for age and gender. At a glance, the slope of her graphed results looked like the Salt Flats in Utah, compared to the Rocky Mountain peaks as indicators of optimal fitness.

She knew her situation before walking in the door. She had hoped that walking out of the club that day would leave her feeling pleased about having a good workout, maybe experiencing a new activity, or making a new acquaintance. Instead, she had a one-hour reminder of how "unfit" or bad she was. It took enormous effort to walk in the door, and it would take even more to come back.

ASSESSING AN INDIVIDUAL'S LEVEL OF FITNESS

Fitness testing can provide information about a person's current level of conditioning and how it compares with national normed data. The information gained from fitness testing can also serve as the basis for determining what can and should be done (e.g., activity and exercise prescriptions) to improve that individual's fitness level. A person's fitness assessment results can also be used as a baseline measure to help them progress toward achieving their exercise- and health-related goals going forward.

On the other hand, is fitness testing always the best option? Arguably, the information is helpful for establishing a baseline and documenting progress. Too much of a focus on numbers and normed comparisons, however, can be discouraging. The fitness assessment data may, at times, be more useful for the trainer than the individual. The information is only useful if it can be communicated in a manner that is accurate, motivating, and positive, since no one feels great about themselves, having just a list of their problems, with no list of solutions.

TRANSFORMING AWARENESS INTO ACTION

Being aware of the importance of a physically active lifestyle is a good beginning. Such an awareness is not sufficient, however. Active participation is necessary in order to receive the benefits of being physically active.

Broadly defined, fitness is considered the ability to engage in activities of daily living without becoming too tired or being injured. Being totally fit refers to the fact that a person has the ability to do the things they need to do and like to do at work, at home, and at play without a heightened risk of injury or undue fatigue. Collectively, fitness is a byproduct of four basic health-related components of fitness—cardiorespiratory fitness, muscular fitness, flexibility, and body composition.

The health-related components of fitness are those factors that impact long-term health. In contrast, the skill-related components of fitness (i.e., motor skills, such as power, agility, coordination, kinesthetic awareness, balance, quickness, and foot speed) are important for performing athletic-type activities, but have little to do with an individual's your long-term health. Total fitness is attained when all four health components are developed and maintained at an appropriate level. Total fitness involves possessing all four fitness elements.

MAKING A COMMITMENT TO CONTINUE BEING PHYSICALLY ACTIVE

If exercise is so beneficial in so many ways, why are the rates of exercise adherence so low? Why do so many people drop out of exercise programs? What (if anything) can be done to increase their level of exercise adherence? Unfortunately, the answers to such questions are not clear cut. Just as people join an exercise program for varying reasons, they may also stop exercising for different reasons. A factor that affects one individual may not be important to another person. Without question, the wide array of potentially influential elements contributing to poor exercise adherence complicates the process of finding all the answers.

In fact, several elements have been identified that have significant impact on exercise adherence, including injuries, time, boredom, and results. Without question, activities that are not "painful" are more enjoyable for most people. Activities that result in discomfort, aches, or injuries are much less so. The old adage, "no pain, no gain," simply doesn't make "sense" to most people.

A number of individuals prefer to engage in exercise regimens that are time-efficient. Time is a valuable resource that is not to be expended wastefully. While some individuals may enjoy exercising aerobically for an hour or more, most people simply don't want to devote that kind of time to such an endeavor. Fortunately, if developing their level of cardiorespiratory fitness is the primary goal of a person's workout, they may only need to exercise continuously for as little as 20 minutes to accomplish that particular exercise objective.

IMPROVING EXERCISE ADHERENCE

Building life-long interest and enjoyment in sport and exercise activities is an essential component of healthy children and adults, as well as the ability of individuals to thrive in an obesogenic culture. Lifelong enjoyment of physical activity is a process that begins in childhood and can be facilitated by parents, teachers, schools, communities, and healthcare providers. The promotion and dissemination of information regarding the benefits of physical activity is critical to having individuals make a lifelong commitment to sustained physical activity.

Parents can help the situation in a number of ways. For example, they can remain positive with regard to their child's involvement in sport. They can also delay initiating their child into the competitive sports arena. Furthermore, they can help "protect" the amount of time their child has for other activities, such as homework and friends. In addition, teachers can have an impact on the effort to protect a child's time for recovery and relaxation. As such, teachers can improve their own level of an awareness concerning what they can and should do to help preserve an individual's motivation and interest in sport. For example, they need to abstain, at all times, from using exercise as punishment.

Schools can also play a role in advancing the value of a physically active lifestyle. For example, they can preserve physical education, recess, and after-school sport activities. Furthermore, they can support building and maintaining safe facilities for those endeavors and activities. In addition, schools can improve access to exercise, team participation and/or physical activity facilities for children of all skills and abilities.

It is absolutely essential that schools discontinue the discriminatory treatment of children who do not test as the most athletic in the school. Sports participation is not just for the 15 kids out of 2000 teens in the school who collectively are the top performers in any particular sport. Sport opportunities should be available to all children and teens, at levels appropriate for their personal skills and interests.

Communities can also be an integral part of the "move-to-improve" pursuit. For example, they can improve safe access for members that they serve to their parks and recreation facilities, as well as maintain their sidewalks and streets in good repair for walking or biking to and from school. Community members and government agencies can also work collaboratively to minimize the impact of any financial strain on exercise and physical activity resources. Furthermore, they can encourage instructors, teachers, and coaches to use respectful, supportive, and caring instructional styles when interacting with the children who reside in their community. Supportive environments can be "hard working," as well as highly successful, environments. To the degree possible, physical activity for children and adults of all sizes should be promoted and assigned value. In addition, individuals and communities can work together to cooperatively and collectively preserve the element of fun in exercise and physical activities in order to improve exercise adherence over a lifetime.

MEETING THE PHYSICAL ACTIVITY "NEEDS" OF THE INDIVIDUAL

Fundamental to any effort to getting people to be physically active on an ongoing basis is making sure that they stick with their exercise regimen. A number of possible steps may be undertaken, in that regard, to enhance the likelihood that an individual's needs will be met by their physical activity efforts, including the following:

- Identify interests in exercise or physical activity programming. Mobility? Health risk reduction? Social connection with others? Lower resting pulse or blood pressure? As such, a person should develop a written list of what they need, want, and expect their exercise efforts to accomplish. Based upon a thorough evaluation of their list (note: the identified needs should be appropriate, clear, and attainable), the individual should develop a strategy that will enable their needs to be met.
- Make exercise fun. If the exercise program isn't enjoyable, the likelihood that a person will stick with it over the long haul is practically nonexistent. Making a program "fun" may require some degree of ingenuity on the exerciser's part. The easiest initial step is to choose an exercise activity that the individual enjoys. If, for example, a person hates to jog, it is simply a waste of their time and efforts to run on a regular basis to try to become more fit. Adding variety to programming can also help. Ensuring that the program offers the exerciser an opportunity for repeated success is another enjoyment-oriented step. One of the primary keys to achieving a successful experience is to focus on pleasure, not pain, in the exercise program.
- Make exercise and physical activity as safe as possible. Moderation is the key. Excess in an individual's exercise program's level of intensity, duration, or frequency can lead to an increase in the number and seriousness of musculoskeletal injuries that they experience. More is not always better with regard to exercise. One key factor for a person is to make sure that they properly use any equipment involved in their exercise regimen. If the exercise program involves the potential of orthopedic trauma (caused by the impact of the feet hitting the floor, for example), the individual should be sure to work out in appropriate footwear. The exerciser should also be sensitive to any existing health-risk factors they might have and to the need to make any resultant program modifications that may be necessary.
- Make programming as effective as possible. Positive results can have a very positive effect on a person's commitment to keep expending the effort necessary to engage in their exercise program. The opposite also holds true. The surest way for an individual to achieve optimal results from their efforts is to base their exercise regimen on sound exercise principles.

- Engage in group activities (if the exerciser enjoys group activities). Research has documented that exercise adherence is lower in programs in which individuals work out by themselves than in those that incorporate group dynamics. For a number of interrelated factors, (which vary from program to program and individual to individual), the social reinforcement, camaraderie, and companionship associated with a group program tend to facilitate a higher level of exercise compliance.

- Set personal program goals for a person who is driven by personal interests and values and periodically assess to what degree their goals are being met. The personal goals of an individual should be mutually developed in consultation between the individual and any certified fitness professional from whom they may solicit advice. The exerciser's goals should be challenging, yet realistic. From time to time, the individual should also assess whether or not their exercise program is working. In other words, the exerciser should periodically evaluate their progress, i.e., determine how effective the program is and whether any adjustments need to be made. It is also important to remember that any physiological or performance results obtained can be used to develop the equivalent of a "report card" to provide the individual with additional positive reinforcement.

- Make program or physical activities convenient and comfortable. Exercise should be scheduled at a time most that is well-matched to the person's schedule of availability (e.g., before work; after work; during the day; etc.). In addition, the area in which the individual exercises should reflect a user-friendly philosophy. The exerciser should also consider working out to music. Research has shown that appropriate background music in an exercise area can be energizing and/or entertaining.

- Solicit support from a close friend or a significant other. The ability to stick with an exercise program is often strongly influenced by how a person's friends or family feel about the individual's involvement with the program. Whenever possible, a person should exercise with other individuals on a regular basis. Their involvement and/or support can improve an exerciser's level of adherence.

ACHIEVING A HEALTHIER TOMORROW

A physically active lifestyle can easily be distinguished from a sedentary one. Fortunately, a healthier tomorrow is well within every individual's reach. The key is making a commitment to be fit. Such an undertaking can be more easily achieved and maintained if the person adopts a commonsense approach to being physically active.

The strategy to be physically active can involve a number of steps, including starting to exercise today (i.e., stop procrastinating); focusing on making relatively small changes over time in your physical activity patterns; exercising with a partner who can help encourage and support your efforts; and making your exercise efforts enjoyable. Another important consideration is to be aware of the fact that your physical activity endeavors don't have to be confined to engaging in a structured exercise regimen. In fact, purposeful movement can occur in a variety of forms, including working in the yard or garden, walking in the neighborhood, shoveling snow, cleaning out the attic, etc. When in doubt, always remember the catchphrase "move to improve." It has relevance for both the quality and the quantity of your life.

The key point is that exercise does not and should not involve drudgery. As such, individuals should not punish themselves if, for whatever reason, they have temporary setbacks in their exercise efforts. Their focus should be to do everything feasible to enhance their level of fitness.

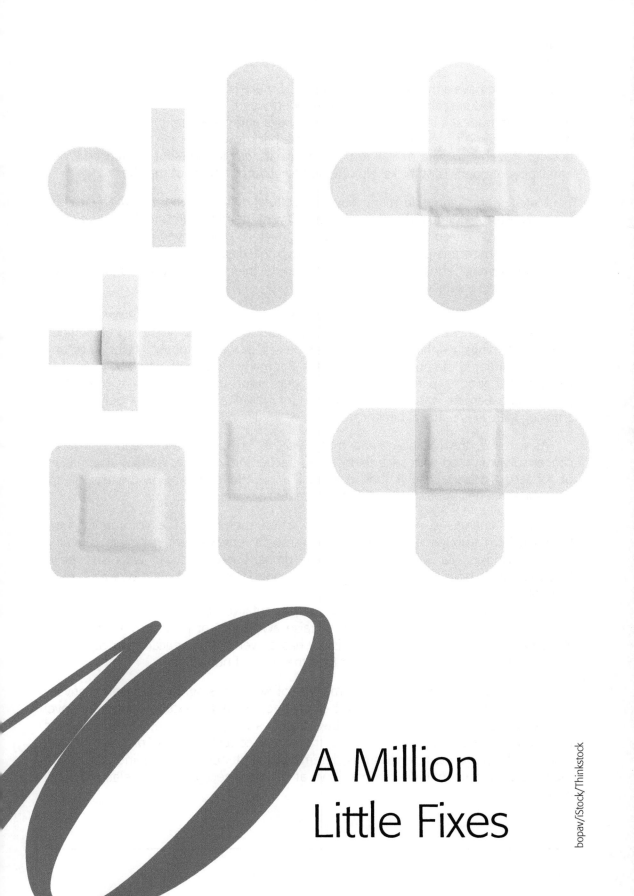

A Million
Little Fixes

"Does anyone have a match?" the Rabbi asked. Smoke curled from the wick of a candle customarily lit during the service. All he needed was a simple match. Of the several hundred attendees, a few rifled through handbags and poked around in their pockets. All but one came up empty-handed. From the back row, a woman passed forward a booklet. Row by row, the miniature parcel made its way to the rabbi. He reached for it and flipped it open. Toothpicks! No one had a lighter or a book of matches.

Matches and lighters in many ways are cultural artifacts of an era when cigarette butts were as ubiquitous as soda cans are today. At the office, around the dining room table, in church parking lots, and even at the doctor's office—even just a half-decade ago—many Americans puffed their way through the day. Reverse the calendar by 30 years, and I imagine that more matchbooks and lighters would have manifested had the rabbi made a similar request.

Since its peak in the mid-1960s, smoking prevalence among Americans has dropped by over 50 percent. Throughout the decades, a steady stream of Surgeon General Warnings, graphic anti-smoking campaigns, as well as tobacco taxes, laws, and litigation, saturated the public consciousness. For many individuals, witnessing the slow demise of a spouse, parent, or friend was persuasion enough. The cost of taking a puff, people learned, was too great a burden for individuals, as well as society, to bear: smoking increases national healthcare costs, while diminishing the life of the smoker.

As a result, the Marlboro man made way for a new smoking icon. A ravaged cancer survivor, fitted with false teeth and a tracheotomy device, warning the masses of tobacco's deadly cost. It took over half a decade of raising awareness of the consequential health hazards, but culture eventually shifted.

Cultural change is possible, especially when members of a community work together. With enough awareness and community engagement, smokers can stop smoking. Drinkers can abstain from driving drunk. Passengers can wear seat belts. Skiers can wear helmets. Voters can pass civil rights laws. After a male college student died of an apparent alcohol related incident in the fraternity house at Virginia State University (November, 2014), a student representative called for "cultural change." Women and men can band together to raise awareness of previously taboo topics, like breast cancer, by wearing pink. History has proven that Americans are capable of change, when the benefits are greater than the costs of not acting.

Immediately following 9/11, the majority of Americans agreed to sacrifice privacy to ensure safety. Therefore, a number of people, to an extent, accepted travel inconveniences at airports, endured bag searches at sporting events, and resigned themselves to Big Brother's oversight of their email correspondence, phone calls, and credit card purchases. If terrorism is deterred, then standing in long lines, taking off their shoes, and submitting to a pat-down at security checkpoints is a relatively small cost to pay.

Cultural shifts have also changed the way individuals parent. Thirty years ago, corporal punishment was an acceptable method for modifying a child's behavior. A child spanked at Target for a tantrum in the toy aisle might have raised a few eyebrows, but not necessarily raised suspicion of a person's parental fitness.

Over time, however, cumulative research has linked corporal punishment to child aggression, antisocial behavior, and delinquency, as well as child abuse and spousal assault later in life. A leading voice in the movement, Dr. Benjamin Spock once remarked, "If we are ever to turn toward a kindlier society and a safer world, a revulsion against the physical punishment of children would be a good place to start." As enraged youth headlined the news, threatening to unleash violence in their homes, schools, parks, theaters, and even churches, culture began to shift.

In the seven decades since the publication of Dr. Spock's internationally renowned book, *Baby and Child Care*, most states have outlawed corporal punishment in schools. One state, Delaware, has even outlawed parental corporal punishment. Though still widely accepted by many parents, corporal punishment is viewed as inappropriate by our culture. Fortunately, a majority of society recognizes that the cost of America's violent youth—loss of life, broken individuals and families that drain the social system, potential legal fees, and even imprisonment—is too great to not apply public pressure and find resolve. With regard to obesity, one of the significant issues is whether our culture can similarly apply pressure to change the trajectory of our national obesity epidemic.

THE HIDDEN COST OF OBESITY

Arguably, the cost of doing nothing is greater than the cost of doing something. From an economic standpoint, America's healthcare system will be drained if the epidemic isn't curbed. According to "F as in Fat: How Obesity Threatens America's Future," released by Trust for America's Health (TFAH) and the Robert Wood Johnson Foundation (RWJF), if obesity rates continue to rise at their current rates, by 2030, in many states obesity will be the new norm. Thirteen states could have adult obesity rates above 60 percent, 39 states could have rates above 50 percent, and all 50 states could have rates above 44 percent.

Between 2010 and 2020, preventable obesity-related diseases, for example, type 2 diabetes, coronary heart disease and stroke, hypertension, and arthritis, could increase 10 times and double again by 2030. These numbers are even more jaw-dropping when they are added to the millions of Americans who already suffer strokes and die from cancer. According to the report:

> *Our healthcare system cannot sustain the costs of these skyrocketing medical conditions, and our economy cannot sustain the lost days of work because of health conditions related to obesity. By 2030, loss in economic productivity could be between $390 billion and $580 billion*

annually. Although the medical cost of adult obesity in the United States is difficult to calculate, current estimates range from $147 billion to nearly $210 billion per year.

Another study calculated the additional healthcare costs of an obese 10-year-old and determined that additional direct medical costs over that particular child's lifetime would mean an additional cost of $20,000. A whopping $14 billion is added to direct U.S. medical costs over the lifetime of currently obese 10-year-olds. Such numbers help quantify the cost of obesity for health insurance companies and government agencies. There are, however, costs that can't easily be mathematically measured.

No one can see the crushed self-esteem or self-loathing of an obese child, alone on the playground, while other children taunt him. No one can see the fear, depression, and anxiety that hound the teenage girl, who, after receiving a "fat letter," turns to bulimia in an attempt to look like either the cover of *Seventeen* magazine or the newest pop sensation. No one can see the despair of the 62-year-old woman who, since her youth, has tried every fad diet but is heavier today than ever. No one can see the dashed hope of the executive, who after losing 100 pounds is asked by peers, "Wow, how much more do you have to lose?"

As a culture, Americans could better understand and appreciate the intricate social-psychological risks that accompany the pursuit of "thin." Our culture applauds thinness and even rewards it with dollars or the cover of a magazine, emphasizing the false notion that extreme thinness is the gateway to success. Blitzed by media messages that "thin" wins and "fat" loses, people are treated differently, based on their size and shape. Weight bias runs deep. On the other hand, it is often unseen and a lot harder to change than a label on a package or a law that modifies vending machines.

Discriminatory behavior is real, however, from the playground to the boardroom. Furthermore, the consequences can be more costly than the medical effects of obesity alone. The American Psychological Association recently declared that emotional abuse can be as malicious as physical abuse or sexual assault.

The "you're-not-good-enough" messages can linger for a lifetime. They can compromise an individual's academics, future livelihood, self-confidence, ability to have relationships, and potential to thrive physically, as well as emotionally. These are example of the hidden costs of the obesity epidemic that can't be quantified by numbers.

The potential consequences of emotional abuse can be dire, including eating disorders, seething self-hatred, chronic despair, or giving up on life completely. To embrace the thin ideal is to also embrace an at-all-costs approach to weight loss that not only overdelivers promises of prosperity, but also compromises the overall mental and physical health of an individual who pursues the thin ideal without ever receiving the crowning reward.

As long as the American culture of fast food, drive-throughs, 32-ounce "to-go" cups, and 24-hour food delivery is accompanied with less and less physical activity and a loathing for people who are obese, the cost of obesity (both emotional and physical) will continue to escalate. As previously stated, obesity is not just a number to be forecasted, charted, and prescribed. It's not merely about cracking the calorie code, through application of more exercise and less food. It's not just a matter of hormone secretion, evolutionary patterns, biology, genetics, neurology, or psychology.

Obesity has been deemed as one disease. *It is not one condition, however.* Obesity is both multiply determined and multiply perpetuated. As such, it must be addressed from multiple directions, with new strategies that look beyond the dial on the scale. What is the professional's role in this endeavor? What is your role as a parent, friend, teacher, scientist, or physician? Is turning a blind eye to the devastating wake created by antiquated strategies the best that can be done? What is each of our individual responsibilities in transcending the destruction that is all too pervasive? What are the possibilities that can be realized in a different future.

The "diet or no diet debate" is not working. The debate entangles great medical and psychological minds, but does not ensure better health. Instead of adopting a unilateral fix, a new approach must appreciate the internal complexities and dangers of thinness at any cost.

At the doctor's office, at school, at the gym, at work, in counseling, and at home, it is time to end the issuance of allegedly ironclad proclamations, such as ideal comparisons, ideal expectations, and telling people who they are and what they should weigh: "You must change;" "You should lose this much weight;" "When you are thin, you will be happy, respected, and healthy." Professionals and their institutions must dial down the dictates and thoughtfully teach, inform, and support people.

Healthcare providers can continue to appreciate the complexity of the obese condition, respect unique and evolving individual needs and interests, provide credible information, and empower individuals to make healthy personal choices. Collective efforts can be increasingly patient-centered and tap the internal resources of individuals and inspire hope, by making such statements as, "What do you value? What do you need? How can I help you?"

As a culture, individuals can avoid assuming that they know how others must manage their health. After a tsunami in Sri Lanka, mental healthcare volunteers traveled from the United States to help the citizens of Sri Lanka cope with the resulting devastation and lost life. Cognitive-behavioral therapy, usual, and customary interventions for trauma were offered. Most Sri Lankans were Buddhist, however. As such, they value existing in their grief and being strong when facing their grief. The cognitive-behavioral techniques were neither appropriate nor successful for that community. As a culture, we can avoid lapsing to the assumptions that limiting caloric intake and expending more energy is the answer for everyone.

Improved health for all people of all sizes—both physical as well as emotional—is hard-earned and incremental. For change to occur, yes, public policy needs to begin to reshape America's obesogenic culture. Yes, healthcare providers and scientists can continue learning how the body works and how best to preserve health. Yes, educators and parents need to teach, model, and provide opportunities for better health. Yes, dieticians and trainers can customize the health plans for their clients. Yes, government and politicians need to consider health and obesity matters in "all" policies, statutes, and laws.

Guiding these changes, however, could be a new framework for approaching weight-related health and weight-related success. A more appropriate approach, one that will actually be more successful, is one that withholds size-related judgment, recognizes each person's unique, and not always, obvious strengths and struggles (e.g., genetic, physiological, socio-economic, cultural, and psychological). A more successful approach will reject perfection and permit setbacks, recognizing that imperfection is inherent to all human experience. As such, a more successful approach will repudiate the practice of pursuing the hypothetical flawless physique. A more successful approach will inspire hope for a future, no matter the number on the scale, recognizing the necessity of personal choice and the value of incremental steps toward better health.

WHERE WE ARE. WHERE WE ARE GOING.

In order to turn the tide of obesity, the tide of childhood obesity must first be addressed. As such, statistics indicate that children who are overweight are likely to be overweight into adulthood. In that regard, more recent research points to the need for early intervention. Kindergartners, for example, who are overweight are more likely to be overweight teens. Heavier youth today translates into a heavier, and possibly a more unhealthy, America tomorrow, with the next generation possibly the first to not outlive their parents. Some experts, though, believe that the situation is far worse. "I think we are going to raise a generation of children that live as long as their parents, but will live with chronic, debilitating diseases that reduce their quality of life," states Professor James Hill, a nutritionist from the University of Colorado.

In late 2013 and early 2014, pockets of sunshine peeked through the deluge of apocalyptic obesity statistics. The Centers for Disease Control first revealed in August 2013 that the obesity trend among low-income preschoolers, ages two to five, dropped in 19 of 43 states and U.S. territories between 2008 and 2011. Six months later, another report was released by the Center for Disease Control that indicated obesity had dropped 43 percent among two- to five-year-olds.

While the rates among other population segments in the study either climbed or leveled off, some individuals hoped that, finally, childhood obesity was on the decline. After all, if children don't enter kindergarten overweight or obese, they statistically are less likely to become overweight in the future. As such, patterns set at an early age persist into adulthood.

Many experts, however, question whether the tide of childhood obesity is truly turning. Are the statistics reliable? A number of experts state that it's too early to know, and more research must be dedicated to understanding what precipitated the drop that has occurred to this point. Was it increased emphasis on nutrition and physical activity in childcare facilities, WIC's (Women, Infant, and Children—a nutrition education food program that helps pregnant and post-partum women, infants, and children under five eat well and stay healthy) emphasis on breastfeeding, or were more parents and teachers restricting the amount of food given to the children? If the latter, then little hope exists that the numbers will stay low. Restrictive eating practices statistically lead to overconsumption, as well as an increased risk for obesity in the future.

The research on childhood obesity is only one broad stroke in the always-developing picture of the obesity epidemic. Just weeks after the hopeful news, researchers from the University of North Carolina reviewed the same study by the CDC and concluded that obesity was worsening, especially among school-aged girls and teenaged boys. Furthermore, the numbers of kids falling in the category of most severely obese appears to be increasing.

Investigative efforts, such as the aforementioned, are why many experts doubt whether the tide has actually begun to turn. David Katz, M.D., director of Yale Prevention and Research, argues that one-in-ten children under five are obese. In reality, excess weight among infants and toddlers hasn't dropped. In other words, the next group of preschoolers to be studied may not show the same downward trajectory.

These statistics are shy of praiseworthy, implies Katz, and are an indication of just "how bad we let things get." Furthermore, the obesity rates among this age group have not fallen steadily, but have been erratic. In some years, the numbers were up, while in other years, the numbers were down. As such, the baseline may not be entirely reliable. According to Katz:

> Here in the U.S., we are, at best, still producing a sizable cohort of obese five-year-olds despite our considerable efforts, and the even larger cohort of obese five-year-olds from several years back is just now entering the age of risk for serious metabolic complications. Here, too, the most severe consequences of rampant childhood obesity [are] yet to come. Here, too, the floodwaters have yet to crest. The lack of change in children under age two looks a bit to me like storm clouds on the horizon.

What can be done to stop the flood waters? Katz offers a provocative metaphor, one that echoes, in some ways, this book's call for culture-wide change. Society, he argues, can hold back the flood water with a levee, built one sandbag at a time. "No one person has to do that all!" he writes. "All anyone needs to do is stack a bag of sand. Stack one bag (or more than one) of sand, and you are part of the solution, and thus not part of the problem. A levee is achieved incrementally—and so, too, can we turn the tide of obesity."

A message posted in the 9/11 memorial in New York City addresses the need for "cooperation" in order to achieve greatness. In that missive, World Trade Center architect, Minoru Yamasaki stated, "Beyond the compelling need to make this a monument to world peace, the World Trade Center should, because of its importance, become a living representation of man's belief in humanity, his need for individual dignity, his beliefs in the cooperation of men, and through this cooperation, his ability to find greatness."

Katz's emphasis on working together is well-taken. No one sandbag can divert the crisis or correct the origin of the flood. In recent years, policymakers, the nonprofit sector, community leaders, educators, healthcare providers, and parents have begun stacking their fair share of sandbags.

The Federal Drug Administration (FDA) is working on restructuring nutrition labels, enlarging the font of the serving size and calories, as well as increasing the serving size, so that they more accurately reflect the actual caloric measure of an item. For instance, ice cream cartons will reflect one-cup servings rather than half-cup servings to account for the amount that a person is more likely to eat. A 2010 federal law health regulation required every chain restaurant to post its calorie information. As part of Obamacare, vending machine providers are required to post calorie counts on vending machines across the country.

In an effort to increase healthful food options in food deserts, the USDA recently passed a farm bill that requires "depth of stock"—more fruits, vegetables, grains, and meats—in convenience stores that are in the Supplemental Nutrition Assistance Program. In turn, the USDA's Healthy Hunger-Free Kids Act incentivizes schools to include more fruits, vegetables, whole grains, and lean meats in their school lunches. "Smart Snacks in Schools," an extension of the Healthy Hunger-Free Kids Act, is an initiative to reinforce healthy choices at school by banning junk food marketing in schools and requiring school vending machines and competitive school vendors to offer only healthful food options.

"CLOCC" (the Consortium to Lower Obesity in Chicago Children) is initiating and organizing various projects that are designed to achieve several goals, including to improve statewide standards for physical activity, nutrition, and screen time for children; to challenge the federal subsidy system that impacts the quality and type of food available to consumers; to incentivize grocers to provide healthy food; to ensure active transportation inclusion in federal legislation promoting safety in physical activity, recreation, and social interaction; to get physical education reinstated into America's schools; and to forge collaboration between schools and healthcare systems. As such, stack upon stack of sandbags, the efforts are mounting.

Local communities are also laying sandbags. Pop-up grocers are setting up mobile grocery stores in food deserts, like Fresh Moves in Chicago, which stocks a retired CTA bus with fresh produce and other items typically not found in convenient stores. Physical fitness programs, like "Girls on the Run," are being introduced in communities to promote health and wellness before and after school. Communities are revamping their built environments, through the support of the Robert Wood Foundation, which provides funding to states through their Safe Routes to School program. Schools are embracing gardening to teach about nutrition and looking for creative ways to incorporate physical activity breaks throughout the day. Consequentially, the number of stacked sandbags seems to rise.

IT DEMANDS INTEGRATION

The sandbag analogy does fall short in a few ways. To prevent flooding, sandbags must be deliberately stacked, each one overlapping another. Furthermore, sandbags are usually a temporary solution to a much bigger problem—where is the water coming from in the first place?

The million little fixes to the obesity epidemic cannot exist in isolation, separate from the other fixes. There is overlap and interactive effects with every intervention, change, or adjustment. Each intervention has ongoing repercussions in culture. There is a reciprocal relationship in all existing and potential changes.

Interventions act on the individual and/or circumstances. In return, the results have an impact on the intervention. Yet, too often, our culture's efforts are isolated and don't work together. In fact, the Trust for America's Health concluded that while obesity initiatives are cropping up, *America lacks the coordination necessary to more successfully address the crisis.*

The efforts to discourage the consumption of junk food in schools are undermined by the cuts in the nation's physical education programs, or by the commonplace elevation of junk food for classroom celebrations illustrate the convoluted nature of the issue. America's agricultural subsidies can also have a negative impact on the situation. For example, in recent years, experts have argued that government-issued subsidies are worsening the obesity epidemic. Subsidizing America's corn crops—the backbone of America's contemporary junk food diet—the USDA toils against the very efforts of their Healthy Hunger-Free Kids Act, which works to eliminate junk from the food choices that schools provide.

The conflicting interests of the USDA can be counterproductive. For example, while improving nutrition in food deserts, a marketing off-shoot of the USDA (Dairy Management) simultaneously partnered with Domino's Pizza to promote a line of pizzas with 40 percent more cheese.* Consumers may have access to more tomatoes

---

*It is important to note that the USDA did not use taxpayer dollars to fund the arrangement between Dairy Management (a marketing organization that targets dairy sales) and Domino's Pizza. This relationship was about the dairy industry paying for marketing services, designed to sell more cheese, that were regulated by the USDA.

and whole grain breads in their nutrition-barren neighborhoods, but they also will be tempted by low-cost, double-the-calorie pizza. To not align efforts is to allow the epidemic to continue seeping into our culture.

The "Let's Move" campaign is another example of likely well-intentioned, but misaligned, efforts. For over four years, the campaign, spearheaded by the First Lady, Michelle Obama, has successfully raised awareness of childhood obesity, focusing on increased activity and healthy food choices, while also lobbying for laws that promote healthier school environments.

In a "Today" show interview, on the fourth anniversary of the "Let's Move" campaign, the First Lady underscored the campaign's mission: "This campaign isn't about how kids look. It's about how kids feel. And, we want our kids to feel, inside, the best that they can feel so that they become all that they were meant to be." But by appearing on "The Biggest Loser" in two consecutive seasons, Mrs. Obama implicitly, and perhaps unintentionally, championed the show's tacit mantra: You win with thin, no matter the emotional and physical cost. Despite good intentions, her message—"It's not about how a person looks but feels"—is undercut.

THE MISSING SANDBAG

After reading Katz's article, a friend asked, "What are the missing sandbags?" and "What part of the levee is most vital?" The questions are one and the same. There is a psychosocial piece to the obesity epidemic that has largely been neglected.

While the cultural strategies for battling weight—e.g., diets and exercise—appear to part of the solution, they are, as argued in this text, actually one of the largest contributors to the obesity epidemic. Obesity is big business for the diet and pharmaceutical industries. For example, diet beverages lead the major market segments of the diet industry by almost 10 times that of the next category (artificial sweeteners). Weight-loss products, books, television shows, marketing, and advertising rake in billions of dollars each year.

While public figures remind everyone that health is about how an individual feels and not what they look like, Americans are bombarded with both subtle and overt promises that a person will be more successful when they have lost weight. Such messages reinforce the antiquated diet mentality with lasting and devastating impact that is far beyond obesity itself.

The traditional diet prescribes the specifics of eating and exercise regimens, which is simply—calories in, calories out. The escalating rates of obesity reflect the failure of this approach. We must engage an approach to weight that evaluates success as more than a number on the scale, BMI chart, or tag in your blue jeans. For a person to take good care of their health and their body is a lifelong journey.

What is weight-related success or what could it be? It may not be what the media, friends, family, or even medical authorities, define as successful. For many individuals, success may be an increased level of mobility, a lower level blood pressure, or better diabetes control. It may be better food control, even when a person's emotions are intense. It might be the ability to ride a roller coaster with their children over summer vacation. It might be playing racquetball or another activity that they abandoned years ago. It could also be just feeling more like yourself. For some, it may mean greater personal acceptance and emotional peace.

Just as varied as people's definition of success, so are the approaches to achieving that success. An approach that targets the behavioral dimensions of overeating permits success to be individually defined, while preserving long-term emotional and physical health. It is vital for individuals to pursue health in a way that is sustainable and free from the emotional and physical vicissitudes of traditional dieting. Establishing reasonable expectations; accepting genetic makeup; recognizing environment influence; knowing what can and can't be changed; comparing yourself with yourself rather than with some ideal; refusing to assign worth to an unsustainable number ... are all more healthy strategies.

A more healthy approach would allow individuals to approach weight-related health in small steps and with mindfulness. It would reduce singular focus on the number of pounds lost or achieving an ideal outcome. That doesn't mean that weight loss isn't achievable. Some individuals will be able to slow their upward weight escalation, and some people will improve their weight stability. Still others may reduce their weight.

Healthy weight can be supported by healthy environments locally, regionally, and nationally that reduce or remove the barriers for success. Healthy environments will support autonomous decisions about health, eating, and exercise. Healthy environments will preserve individual motivation over time. A healthy environment will respect individuals of all sizes and their individual decisions about their body, exercise, and eating.

Americans can look beyond the traditional diet. Weight isn't about the gym and restricting foods. For the single mom, working double shifts, driving to a gym for a kickboxing class three times a week, for example, is, frankly, unrealistic. On the other hand, what if during the spare time she has with her children, she walks with them to a park, goes on a bike ride, or takes the kids ice skating at a public rink? For some families and individuals, working out at the gym is enjoyable and economically feasible. A healthy approach is about determining the situation that provides the greatest enjoyment and reward, so that participating in a chosen activity is enjoyable and sustainable for a lifetime of good health.

MOVING FORWARD

- Highlight holistic health perspectives.
- Consider immediate and long term outcome for all interventions.

- Approach choices regarding food and exercise with flexibility and mindfulness.
- Harness internal motivation for better self-care.
- Understand the broader cultural context within which obesity exists.
- Apply current knowledge to improve the overall human condition.
- Apply current knowledge for diverse populations, i.e., age, gender, race, and ethnicity.

ARE WE READY?

Redefining success as something different than "pounds lost" is a cultural shift for which many individuals are not ready. In reality, most people can't remember when they first believed "fat" was bad; the message has been ever-present and pervasive. From Barbie dolls to comic book heroes, individuals have learned to fear flab more than death. Recently, a self-professed "plus-size" teen, Jewel Moore started a petition, requesting Disney to produce positive plus-size protagonists—someone as "bright, amazing, and memorable as their others."

A month later, Moore argued her case on the "Today" show, during which a response from Disney was read: "There are many types of princesses, just as there are many types of girls, who each have their own unique history, character, and story. We appreciate and celebrate all types of women and girls and their own individual beauty."

Brave, a Disney movie released in 2012, broke the princess mold when it featured a heroine with red hair. Time will tell if the appreciation of "individual beauty" will apply to a shape other than thin. Culture may not be ready for such a shift.

Society may not be ready for a shift in which people of different shapes and sizes are embraced. Such an alteration in attitude may be as difficult as many individuals perceive weight loss itself to be. Somehow as a society, we were able to see equality between blacks and whites; we were able to move from a homophobic society to one that has embraced same sex marriages even being supported by the Supreme Court; and we were able to embrace our strength as a country in our melting pot of diversity, rather than limit ourselves to only one color, one language, and one place of birth.

We are strong because we accept differences—we are not weakened by them. Embracing that which is familiar—"Fat is bad, so lose it all"—is far easier. It takes courage to not assign worth to weight and accept the reality that the human body is not infinitely malleable. In addition to a person's genetics, biology, culture, economics, family structures, and emotional health can complicate weight loss.

Culture's pervasive weight-related stigma interferes with the ability to consider and accept higher body weight as healthy or embrace more modest weight loss. If culture learned to respect the limitations of the human body; to appreciate the process rather than the end result; to recognize the medical, social, and psychological risks associated with dieting behavior; and to define success beyond BMI, then arguably, our responses to those who are obese could also change.

We would no longer punish people who are overweight by making them take "fat" gym classes. We would no longer shame kids because of their BMI. We would no longer judge the overweight individual on the treadmill at the gym. We would no longer show preferential treatment toward slimmer students in learning environments. We would no longer dismiss obese patients' medical concerns that are unrelated to weight. We would no longer associate obesity with laziness, and would, consequently, spend less time with obese patients than "normal" size patients. We would no longer punish people for being who they are.

Unfortunately, culture is often more focused on changing circumstances of the past than creating hope and possibilities for the future. It is the rarity to find communities working together to create environments that are conducive to sustaining wellness and weight far into the future. Change is not impossible, however. One way to overcome the impossible is to alter the climate that sustains the impossible, thereby permitting constructive change for a healthier future.

How difficult is the problem for the average American? If only a small segment of healthcare professionals can articulate the magnitude of entry and touch points that affect obesity and realize how expansive the mission will need to be in changing how our culture thinks about obesity and weight loss success, then how can the average American be expected to make informed decisions on what is best for them?

In that regard, some individuals think about health improvements, while others are concerned with risk prevention. Unfortunately, a relatively large number of poseurs are concerned with the profits amassed at the expense of other people's health. In reality, pharmaceutical companies, the fast food industry, eating disorder treatment facilities, diet products companies, and the soft drink industry all profit from obesity. Those individuals most inclined to embrace a cultural change are those who have witnessed the devastation of obesity and eating disorders—parents, friends, behavioral health professionals, school counselors, teachers, dieticians, and doctors.

Imagine if this segment of the population began to accept a new model of weight loss and the impact it would have on culture at large. What if children learned to accept their shape and weren't forced into endless diets that too often resulted in eating disorders or unhealthy weight gain? What if parents learned, early on, to dialogue with their children about health, diversity of size, and faulty cultural models of success? What if parents modeled healthier self-care and rejected the notion of perfection? What if individuals stopped envisioning foods as good or bad and instead taught themselves and their children to approach food mindfully? What if physical activity was not something a person had to do but wanted to do? What if judgments about weight were withheld? What if people were rewarded for healthy behaviors, rather than punished for their weight? What if more doctors inspired hope? What if doctors regarded the "person" more and the "box to check" less? What if the available education dollars were invested in more opportunities for physical fitness and health awareness? What if schools refused to tolerate weightism and bullying? What if companies were able to profit from truly supporting improved health by providing products that were reliable and valid, rather than selling products having no chance in assisting the individual and worse may damage health?

I was recently called into a therapeutic dining session, one in which staff worked hard to sooth and support a distraught patient. She had been restricting food for over one year. She had lost 30 percent of her body weight. She had been discharged with no improvement from two other treatment facilities. She knew that if her weight-loss pattern did not change soon, she would need to reenter the hospital or die.

Our most kind, patient, and thoughtful dietitians were encouraging, reminding, listening, and reassuring. She begged to not eat. She was terrified of weight gain. She felt that it would wipe out everything she had been working toward over the last year. She cried. "Please," she implored. "Don't make me eat."

I sat down across from her, close and making sure that my eyes were level with hers. I listened to her describe her fears, her frustrations, her despair. After several minutes of listening, I told her that I could hear her tremendous fear about eating, weight gain, and fat. I then asked her what else she really most wanted for herself; without pause she answered, "I just want to be understood."

A TIME FOR CHANGE

We are all different shapes and sizes but we are also all more alike than different. The anecdotal stories presented in this book are just a few of the million strategies that have the potential to change the obesity epidemic. While no one simple solution exists to obesity, there are simple steps that each of us can take. Each simple step contributes to the whole and to the change that needs to sweep our country for an *"UnWeighted Nation."*

APPENDIX A
SUGGESTED REFERENCES

2012 IFIC Foundation Food & Health Survey Media Resources. (2012, May 22). *Food Insights*. From http://www.foodinsight.org/2012_IFIC_Foundation_Food_Health_Survey_Media_Resources

2012 Shape of the Nation Report: Quick Facts. (2012). *National Association for Sport and Physical Education & American Heart Association*. From http://www.shapeamerica.org/advocacy/son/2012/upload/2012-shape-of-nation-full-report-web.pdf

Access to Affordable and Nutritious Food: Measuring and Understanding Food Deserts and Their Consequences. (2009, June). *USDA, 1-160*. From http://www.ers.usda.gov/media/242675/ap036_1_.pdf

Ahmed, S. H., Kenny, P. J., Koob, G. F., & Markou, A. (2002, July 10). Neurobiological evidence for hedonic allostasis associated with escalating cocaine use. *Nat. Neurosci. Nature Neuroscience*. doi:10.1038/nn872

Alderman, L. (2010, November 05). Putting Nutrition at the Head of the School Lunch Line. *The New York Times*. From http://www.nytimes.com/2010/11/06/health/06patient.html?_r=0

Alfaris, N., Kyle, T.K., Nadai, J. & Stanford, F.C. (2016, June 21). A New Era Of Addiction Treatment Amplifies The Stigma And Treatment For Individuals With Obesity. *International Journal of Obesity*. 40:1335-1536. doi: 10.1038/ijo. 2016. 101

American Time Use Survey Summery. (2013, June 20). *Bureau of Labor Statistics*. From http://www.bls.gov/news.release/atus.nr0.htm

Anderson, J. (2008). 6 "Biggest Loser" Lessons to Unlearn. From http://www.sparkpeople.com/resource/motivation_articles.asp?id=1192

Anderson, P. M., & Butcher, K. F. (2006). Childhood Obesity: Trends and Potential Causes. *The Future of Children*, 16(1), 19-45. doi:10.1353/foc.2006.0001

Anderson, P. M., & Butcher, K. F. (2006). Reading, Writing, and Refreshments. *Journal of Human Resources J. Human Resources*, XLI(3), 467-494. doi:10.3368/jhr.xli.3.467

Anderson, P., Butcher, K., & Schanzenbach, D. W. (2011, March). Adequate (or Adipose?) Yearly Progress: Assessing the Effect of "No Child Left Behind" on Children's Obesity. *National Bureau of Economic Research*. doi:10.3386/w16873

Anderson, S. (1990). Core indicators of nutritional state for difficult to sample populations. *Journal of Nutrition*, 102(suppl 11), 1559-1660.

Atkin, A. J., Gorely, T., Biddle, S. J., Marshall, S. J., & Cameron, N. (2008, November). Critical Hours: Physical Activity and Sedentary Behavior of Adolescents after School. *Pediatric Exercise Science*, 20(4), 446-456. doi:10.1123/pes.20.4.446

Bamford, B., & Sly, R. (2010, December 2). Exploring quality of life in the eating disorders. *European Eating Disorders Review Eur. Eat. Disorders Rev.*, 18(2), 147-153. doi:10.1002/erv.975

Bauer, K. W., MacLehose, R., Loth, K. A., Fisher, J. O., Larson, N. I., Neumark-Sztainer, D. (2015, September). Eating- and weight-related parenting of adolescents in the context of food insecurity. *Journal of the Academy of Nutrition and Dietetics,* 115(9), 1408-1416.

Bell, J.A., Shipley, M.J., & Kivimaki, M. (2016, May 24). Healthy Obesity Is Not Safe Obesity. *International Journal of Obesity*. 40:1333. doi: 10.1038/ijo. 2016. 77

Bhasin, K. (2013, August 2). Lululemon Admits Plus-Size Clothing Is Not Part Of Its 'Formula'. From http://www.huffingtonpost.com/2013/08/02/lululemon-plus-size-clothing_n_3696690.html

Bieghle, A. (2012, January 01). *Robert Wood Johnson Foundation*. From www.rwjf.org

Boone, J. E., Gordon-Larsen, P., Adair, L. S., & Popkin, B. M. (2007, June 8). Screen time and physical activity during adolescence: Longitudinal effects on obesity in young adulthood. *International Journal of Behavioral Nutrition and Physical Activity*, 4(1), 26. doi:10.1186/1479-5868-4-26

Botha, S., Fentonmiller, K., Jennings, C., Johnson, M., Rusk, M.K., Young, K., et al. (2012, December). A Review of Food Marketing to Children and Adolescents: Follow-Up Report. Washington D.C: Federal Trade Commission. From https://www.ftc.gov/sites/default/files/documents/reports/review-food-marketing-children-and-adolescents-follow-report/121221foodmarketingreport.pdf

Bouchard, C., & Katzmarzyk, P. T. (2010). Physical Activity and Obesity (2nd ed.). Champaign, IL: Human Kinetics.

Boutelle, K., Fulkerson, J. A., Neumark-Sztainer, D., & Story, M. (2004, November). Mothers' Perceptions of Their Adolescents' Weight Status: Are They Accurate? *Obesity Research*, 12(11), 1754-1757. doi:10.1038/oby.2004.217

Bray, G. A. (2016, September). Weight management and exercise: any advantage? *American Journal of Clinical Nutrition*, 104(3), 547-548.

Brown, B. (2012). *Daring Greatly: How the Courage to be Vulnerable Transforms the Way We Live, Love, Parent, and Lead.* New York, NY: Gotham Books.

Brown, H. (2013, January 09). Feeling Bullied by Parents About Weight. From http://well. blogs.nytimes.com/2013/01/09/feeling-bullied-by-parents-about-weight/?_r=0

Brown, M. T., & Bussell, J. K. (2011, April). Medication Adherence: WHO Cares? *Mayo Clinic Proceedings*, 86(4), 304-314. doi:10.4065/mcp.2010.0575

Brownell, K. D. (1991). Dieting and the search for the perfect body: Where physiology and culture collide. *Behavior Therapy*, 22(1), 1-12. doi:10.1016/s0005-7894(05)80239-4

Brownell, K. D. (1991). Dieting and the search for the perfect body: Where physiology and culture collide. *Behavior Therapy*, 22(1), 1-12. doi:10.1016/s0005-7894(05)80239-4

Brownell, K. D. (1991). Dieting and the search for the perfect body: Where physiology and culture collide. *Behavior Therapy*, 22(1), 1-12. doi:10.1016/s0005-7894(05)80239-4

Burleigh, N. (2012). Rahm 2.0. *Du Jour*; 188-193. From http://issue.com/maxmcd/docs/dujour-winter/192

Caleyachetty, R., Meunning, P., & Kengne, A.P. (2016, May 17). Misclassification of cardiometabolic health when using body mass index categories. *International Journal of Obesity*. 40:1332. doi:10.1038/ijo. 2016. 65

Callahan, D. (2012, December 18). Obesity: Chasing an Elusive Epidemic. *Hastings Center Report*, 43(1), 34-40. doi:10.1002/hast.114

Cheung, P. C., Cunningham, S. A., Narayan, K. V., & Kramer, M. R. (2016). Childhood Obesity Incidence in the United States: A Systematic Review. *Childhood Obesity*, *12*(1), 1-11. doi:10.1089/chi.2015.0055

Ciganek, W. & Conviser, J. (2012, August). Treating the Obese Patient. *Chicago Medicine*. From www.cmsdocs.org.

Class of 2015, How They Will Learn and What They Will Pay? (2013, October 7). *Time*. 40-44.

Clinical guidelines on the identification, evaluation, and treatment of overweight and obesity in adults: The evidence report. (1998, September). *National Heart, Lung, and Blood Institute*. Bethesda, MD: National Institute of Health. doi:10.1037/e565682010-001

Clinical guidelines on the identification, evaluation, and treatment of overweight and obesity in adults: The evidence report. (1998, September). *National Heart, Lung, and Blood Institute*. doi:10.1037/e565682010-001

Coleman-Jensen, A., Nord, M., Andrews, M., Carlson, S. (2011, September). Household Food Security in the United States, 2010. Economic Research Report No. (ERR-125). Washington, DC: US Department of Agriculture, Economic Research Division.

Collingwood, J. (2014, March 27). Obesity and Mental Health. *Psych Central*. From http://psychcentral.com/lib/obesity-and-mental-health/

Confronting bias against obese patients. (2013, September 2). *Amednews.com*. From http://www.*amednews.com*/article/20130902/profession/130909988/4/

Corwin, R. L., Avena, N. M., & Boggiano, M. M. (2011, July 25). Feeding and reward: Perspectives from three rat models of binge eating. *Physiology & Behavior, 104*(1), 87-97. doi:10.1016/j.physbeh.2011.04.041

Cote, J., & Hay, J. (2002). Children's Involvement in Sport: A Developmental Perspective. In J. M. Silva, & D. E Stevens (Eds.). *Psychological Foundations of Sport* (pp. 484-502). Boston: Allyn & Bacon.

Cramer, P., & Steinwert, T. (1998). Thin is good, fat is bad: How early does it begin? *Journal of Applied Developmental Psychology, 19*(3), 429-451. doi:10.1016/s0193-3973(99)80049-5

Crosnoe, R. (2007, July). Gender, Obesity, and Education. *Sociology of Education, 80*(3), 241-260.

Crosnoe, R. (2007, July). Gender, Obesity, and Education. *Sociology of Education, 80*(3), 241-260.

Currie, J. (2008, May). Healthy, Wealthy, and Wise: Socioeconomic Status, Poor Health in Childhood, and Human Capital Development. *Journal of Economic Literature, 47*(1), 87-122. doi:10.3386/w13987

Dallas, M. E. (2013, May 31). Obese Patients May Be More Prone to 'Doctor Shopping'. *HealthDay*. From https://consumer.*healthday*.com/general-health-information-16/doctor-news-206/obese-patients-may-be-more-prone-to-doctor-shopping-676633.html

Danaei, G., Ding, E. L., Mozaffarian, D., Taylor, B., Rehm, J., Murray, C. J., & Ezzati, M. (2011, January 10). Correction: The Preventable Causes of Death in the United States: Comparative Risk Assessment of Dietary, Lifestyle, and Metabolic Risk Factors. *PLoS Med PLoS Medicine*, 8(1). doi:10.1371/annotation/0ef47acd-9dcc-4296-a897-872d182cde57

Davison, K. K., & Birch, L. L. (2001, January 01). Weight Status, Parent Reaction, and Self-Concept in Five-Year-Old Girls. *Pediatrics, 107*(1), 46-53. doi:10.1542/peds.107.1.46

Dennison, B. A., Erb, T. A., & Jenkins, P. L. (2002, June 01). Television Viewing and Television in Bedroom Associated With Overweight Risk Among Low-Income Preschool Children. *Pediatrics, 109*(6), 1028-1035. doi:10.1542/peds.109.6.1028

Després, J. P. (2015, December). Exercise and energy balance: going to extremes to show that body weight is not the best outcome. *American Journal of Clinical Nutrition*, 102(6), 1303-1304.

Diet, Nutrition and the prevention of chronic diseases. (2002). *World Health Organization*.

Diez, W. H. (1998, March). Health Consequences of Obesity in Youth: Childhood Predictors of Adult Disease. *Pediatrics, 101*.

Dishman, R. K., Heath, G., & Lee, I. (2013). *Physical Activity Epidemiology*. Champaign, IL: Human Kinetics.

Doctor refuses to treat overweight Shrewsbury patient. (2012, August 24). *WCVB*. From http://www.wcvb.com/health/Doctor-refuses-to-treat-overweight-Shrewsbury-patient/16255838

Donnelly, J. E., Blair, S. N., Jakicic, J. M., Manore, M. M., Rankin, J. W., & Smith, B. K. (2009, July). Appropriate Physical Activity Intervention Strategies for Weight Loss and Prevention of Weight Regain for Adults. *Medicine & Science in Sports & Exercise, 41*(2), 459-471. doi:10.1249/mss.0b013e3181949333

Downey, M. (2013, February 7). The Wage Penalty and Obesity. *Downey Obesity Report*. From http://www.downeyobesityreport.com/2013/02/the-wage-penalty-and-obesity/

Duda, J. L., & Ntoumanis, N. (2005). After-School Sport for Children: Implications of a Task-Involving Motivational Climate. In J. I. Mahoney, R. Larson, & J. Eccles (Eds.) *Organized Activities as Context of Development: Extracurricular Activities, After-School and Community Programs* (pp. 311-330). Mahwah, NJ: Erlbaum.

Educating the Student Body: Taking Physical Activity and Physical Education to School. (2013, May 23). *NASEM*. doi:10.17226/18314

Edwards, K. (2013, June 24). When Your Mother Says She's Fat. *Role Reboot*. From http://www.rolereboot.org/life/details/2013-06-when-your-mother-says-shes-fat

Ervin, R. B. & Ogden, C. L. (2013, February). Trends in intake of energy and macronutrients in children and adolescents from 1999-2000 through 2009-2010. *NCHS Data Brief*. From http://www.cdc.gov/nchs/data/databriefs/db113.pdf

Ervin, R. B., Kit, B. K., Carroll, M. D. & Ogden, C. L. (2012, February). Consumption of Added Sugar Among U.S. Children and Adolescents, 2005–2008. *Centers for Disease Control and Prevention*. From http://www.cdc.gov/nchs/data/databriefs/db87.htm#findings

Ewing, M. E., & Seefeldt, V. (1989). *Participation and Attrition Patterns in American Agency-sponsored and Interscholastic Sports: An Executive Summery.* North Palm Beach, FL: Sporting Goods Manufacturing Association.

F as in Fat: How Obesity Threatens America's Future 2012. (2012, September). *Trust for America's Health.* From http://healthyamericans.org/report/100/

Faber, A., Mazlish, E., Nyberg, L., & Templeton, R. A. (1996). *How To Talk So Kids Can Learn at Home and at School.* New York, NY: Simon and Schuster.

Facts & Statistics. *President's Council on Fitness, Sports & Nutrition.* From http://www.fitness.gov/resource-center/facts-and-statistics/

Fairfield, H. (2010, April 03). Factory Food. *The New York Times.* From http://www.nytimes.com/2010/04/04/business/04metrics.html

Farrow, C. V., Haycraft, E., Blissett, J. M. (2015, May). Teaching our children when to eat: how parental feeding practices inform the development of emotional eating—a longitudinal experimental design. *American Journal of Clinical Nutrition,* 101(5), 908-913.

Fast Food Eating Statistics. (2014, January 1). *Statistic Brain.* From http://www.statisticbrain.com/fast-food-statistics/

Fat letter in public schools. (2013). *The American Academy of Pediatrics.*

Finer, N. (2015, January 28). Predicting therapeutic weight loss. *American Journal of Clinical Nutrition.* 101:419-420. doi: 10.3945/ajcn. 114. 106195

Finkelstein, D. M., Hill, E. L., & Whitaker, R. C. (2008, July). School Food Environments and Policies in US Public Schools. *Pediatrics, 122*(1), 251-259. doi:10.1542/peds.2007-2814

Fitzgibbon, M. L., & Beech, B. M. (2009, September). The Role of Culture in the Context of School-Based BMI Screening. *Pediatrics, 124*, 50-62. doi:10.1542/peds.2008-3586h

Flam, L. (2014, February 28). Teen circulates petition for plus-size princess. *TODAY.* From http://www.*today*.com/health/teen-circulates-petition-plus-size-princess-2D79298377

Foster, G. D., Wadden, T. A., Makris, A. P., Davidson, D., Sanderson, R. S., Allison, D. B., & Kessler, A. (2003, October). Primary Care Physicians' Attitudes About Obesity and Its Treatment. *Obesity Research, 11*(10), 1168-1177. doi:10.1038/oby.2003.161

Francis, L. A., Birch, L. L. (2005). Maternal weight status modulates the effects of restriction on daughters eating and weight. *International Journal of Obesity,* 29(8), 942-949.

Franck, C., Grandi, S. M., & Eisenberg, M. J. (2013). Agricultural Subsidies and the American Obesity Epidemic. *American Journal of Preventive Medicine, 45*(3), 327-333. doi:10.1016/j.amepre.2013.04.010

Fraser-Thomas, J. L., Côté, J., & Deakin, J. (2005, February). Youth sport programs: An avenue to foster positive youth development. *Physical Education & Sport Pedagogy, 10*(1), 19-40. doi:10.1080/1740898042000334890

Freedman, D. (2013, July/August). How Junk Food Can End Obesity. *The Atlantic.* From http://www.theatlantic.com/magazine/archive/2013/07/how-junk-food-can-end-obesity/309396/

Freeman, D. (2011, May 17). Fat-phobic doctors refuse to treat obese patients: Is that fair? *CBS News.* From http://www.cbsnews.com/news/fat-phobic-doctors-refuse-to-treat-obese-patients-is-that-fair/

Fuel Up to Play 60. From http://school.fuelltoplay60.com

Fung T. T., Long, M. W., Hung, P., Cheung, L. W. (2016, July). An expanded model for mindful eating for health promotion and sustainability: issues and challenges for dietetics practice. *Journal of the Academy of Nutrition and Dietetics, 116*(7), 1081-1086.

Fusco, M. (2016). 5 Experts on "The Biggest Loser". Gastric Bypass. From http://doctorsofweightloss.com/5-experts-on-the-biggest-loser

Gallup. (2010, February 01). The State of Play. *Robert Wood Johnson Foundation.* From http://www.rwjf.org/en/library/research/2010/02/the-state-of-play.html

Geier, A. B., Foster, G. D., Womble, L. G., Mclaughlin, J., Borradaile, K. E., Nachmani, J., . . . Shults, J. (2007, August). The Relationship Between Relative Weight and School Attendance Among Elementary Schoolchildren. *Obesity, 15*(8), 2157-2161. doi:10.1038/oby.2007.256

Gilbert, E. D. (2001, October). Towards a Richer Understanding of Girls' Sport Experiences. *Women in Sport and Physical Activity Journal, 10*(2), 117-143. doi:10.1123/wspaj.10.2.117

Global status report on noncommunicable diseases 2010. (2010). *World Health Organization, 161.* From http://www.who.int/nmh/publications/ncd_report_full_en.pdf

Gould, D., & Petlichkoff, L. (1982). Participation motivation and attrition in young athletes. In R. A. Magill, M. J. Ash, & F. L. Smoll, (Eds.). *Children in sport* (3rd ed., pp. 161-178). Champaign, IL: Human Kinetics.

Greenway, F.L. (2015, May 26). Physiological adaptations to weight loss and factors favouring weight regain. *International Journal of Obesity*. 39:1188-1196; doi:10.1038/ijo.2015.59

Gudzune, K. A., Bleich, S. N., Richards, T. M., Weiner, J. P., Hodges, K., & Clark, J. M. (2013, July 13). Doctor shopping by overweight and obese patients is associated with increased healthcare utilization. *Obesity, 21*(7), 1328-1334. doi:10.1002/oby.20189

Guo, Q., Ma, W., Nie, S., Xu, Y., Xu, H., & Zhang, Y. (2010, May 18). Relationships Between Weight Status and Bullying Victimization among School-aged Adolescents in Guangdong Province of China. *Biomedical and Environmental Sciences, 23*(2), 108-112.

Haines, J., Neumark-Sztainer, D., Hannan, P. J., Berg, P. V., & Eisenberg, M. E. (2008, November). Longitudinal and Secular Trends in Weight-related Teasing during Adolescence. *Obesity, 16*(Suppl 2), S18-S23. doi:10.1038/oby.2008.447

Hamblin, J. (2013, October 30). In Lieu of Candy, Woman Handing Out This Letter That Says Child Is Fat. *The Atlantic*. From http://www.theatlantic.com/health/archive/2013/10/in-lieu-of-candy-woman-handing-out-this-letter-that-says-child-is-fat/281002/

Harrington, S. (n.d). The Case for Organizational Culture Change. *Recovery Academy*. From http://webs.wichita.edu/depttools/depttoolsmemberfiles/ccsr/TIC/Case%20for%20Org%20%20Change_Steve%20Harrington.pdf

Harris, J. L., Bargh, J. A., & Brownell, K. D. (2009, July). Priming effects of television food advertising on eating behavior. *Health Psychology, 28*(4), 404-413. doi:10.1037/a0014399

Harris, J. L., Bargh, J.A., & Brownwell, K.D (2009). Priming effects of television food advertising on eating behavior. *Health Psychology* 28: 404-413.

Healy, M. (2013, August 15). Obesity's death toll could be higher than believed, study says. Los Angeles Times. From http://articles.latimes.com/2013/aug/15/science/la-sci-obesity-20130816

Hecimovich, M. (2004). Sport specialization in youth: a literature review. *Journal of the American Chiropractic Association*, 41, (4), 32-41.

Hedstrom, R. & Gould, D. (2004). Research in Youth Sports: Critical Issues Status. Unpublished manuscript, Michigan State University, East Lansing.

Hendrick, B. (2011, April 14). Most Young Kids Don't Get Enough Exercise. *WebMD*. From http://www.*webmd*.com/children/news/20110414/most-young-kids-dont-get-enough-exercise#1

Hetter, K. (2012, March 16). Fat is the new ugly on the playground. CNN. From http://www.cnn.com/2012/03/16/living/body-image-kids/

Heuer, C. A. (2016). *Obesity Action Coalition* » "Fattertainment" – Obesity in the Media. *Obesity Action Coalition*. From http://www.obesityaction.org/educational-resources/resource-articles-2/weight-bias/fattertainment-obesity-in-the-media

Ho, S. (2013, May 11). Students split on Prospect High's divided PE curriculum. *Chicago Tribune*. From http://articles.chicagotribune.com/2013-05-11/news/ct-met-fat-gym-20130511_1_fitness-test-students-fitness-levels

Hood, M. Y., Moore, L. L., Sundarajan-Ramamurti, A., Singer, M., Cupples, L. A., & Ellison, R. C. (2000). Parental eating attitudes and the development of obesity in children. The Framingham Children's Study. *Int J Obes Relat Metab Disord International Journal of Obesity, 24*(10), 1319-1325. doi:10.1038/sj.ijo.0801396

How Americans Eat *Today*. (2010, January 12). *CBS News*. From http://www.cbsnews.com/news/how-americans-eat-*today*/

How Children Get to School: School Travel Patterns from 1969 to 2009. (2011). *The National Center for Safe Routes to School*. From http://www.saferoutesinfo.org/program-tools/NHTS-school-travel-1969-2009

http://www.slideshare.net/jonlar/the-us-weight-loss-market-in-2013

http://www.wfmj.com/story/25180211/childhood-obesity-adds-nearly-20k-to-lifetime-medical-costs-study

Huizinga, M. M., Cooper, L. A., Bleich, S. N., Clark, J. M., & Beach, M. C. (2009, September 18). Physician Respect for Patients with Obesity. *Journal of General Internal Medicine,* 24(11), 1236-1239.

Jameson, M. (2011, July 04). Restaurants obesity: Eating at restaurants boosts risk of obesity, experts warn. *Orlando Sentinel*. From http://articles.orlandosentinel.com/2011-07-04/health/os-restaurants-obesity-20110704_1_restaurant-foods-eating-obesity-experts

Janssen, I., Craig, W. M., Boyce, W. F., & Pickett, W. (2004, May). Associations Between Overweight and Obesity With Bullying Behaviors in School-Aged Children. *Pediatrics, 113*(5), 1187-1194. doi:10.1542/peds.113.5.1187

Jaslow, R. (2013, November 20). Kids less physically fit than parents were at their age. *CBS News*. From http://www.cbsnews.com/news/kids-less-physically-fit-than-parents-were-at-their-age/

Jennifer Lawrence: Quotes. (n.d.). From http://m.imdb.com/name/nm2225369/quotes

Jess. (2011, October 10). *xoJane*. From http://www.*xojane*.com/healthy/dear-doctors-quit-it-weight-bullying

Kam, K. (2010). The Facts on Leptin: FAQ - The truth about the hormone leptin and obesity. *WebMD*. From http://www.*webmd*.com/diet/obesity/features/the-facts-on-leptin-faq#1

Kark, M., & Karnehed, N. (2012, September 28). Weight status at age 18 influences marriage prospects. A population-based study of Swedish men. *BMC Public Health, 12*(1), 833. doi:10.1186/1471-2458-12-833

Katz, M. D. (2012, May 19). Obesity, Be Dammed! The *Huffington Post*. From http://www.huffingtonpost.com/david-katz-md/obesity_b_1527695.html

Kelner, K., & Helmuth, L. (2003, February 07). Obesity-What Is To Be Done? *Science, 299*(4), 845-845. doi:10.1126/science.299.5608.845

Kirk, D. (2005, October). Physical education, youth sport and lifelong participation: The importance of early learning experiences. *European Physical Education Review, 11*(3), 239-255. doi:10.1177/1356336x05056649

Kral, I. G., Sjostrom, L. V. & Sullivan. M. B. E. (1992, February). Assessment of quality of life before and after surgery for severe obesity. *American Journal of Clinical Nutrition, 55, 611-614*.

Krukowski, R., West, D. S., Perez, A. P., Bursac, Z., Phillips, M., & Raczynski, J. (2009, November 18). Overweight children, weight-based teasing and academic performance. *Int. J. of Pediatric Obesity SPOB International Journal of Pediatric Obesity, 4*(4), 274-280. doi:10.1080/17477160902846203

Kubik, M. Y., Davey, C., MacLehose, R. F., Coombes, B., Nanney, M. S. (2015, January). Snacks, beverages, vending machines, and school stores: a comparison of alternative and regular schools in Minnesota, 2002 to 2008. *Journal of the Academy of Nutrition and Dietetics,* 115(1), 101-105.

La Rosa, J. (2013, November 06). Overview and statistics of the U.S weight loss market.

Lagisz, M. Blair, H., Kenyon, P.,Uller, T., Raubenheiner, D., & Nakagawa. S.

(2015, September 15). Little appetite for obesity: meta-analysis of the effects of material obesogenic diets on offspring food intake and body mass in rodents. *International Journal of Obesity*. 39:1669-1678; doi:10.1038/ijo.2015.160

Landhuis, C. E., Poulton, R., Welch, D., & Hancox, R. J. (2008, June 27). Programming Obesity and Poor Fitness: The Long-term Impact of Childhood Television. *Obesity, 16*(6), 1457-1459. doi:10.1038/oby.2008.205

Lemyre, P., Hall, H. K., & Roberts, G. C. (2007, July 09). A social cognitive approach to burnout in elite athletes. *Scandinavian Journal of Medicine & Science in Sports, 18*(2), 221-234. doi:10.1111/j.1600-0838.2007.00671.x

Li, S., Zhao, J. H., Luan, J., Ekelund, U., Luben, R. N., Khaw, K., . . . Loos, R. J. (2010, August 31). Physical Activity Attenuates the Genetic Predisposition to Obesity in 20,000 Men and Women from EPIC-Norfolk Prospective Population Study. *PLoS Med PLoS Medicine, 7*(8). doi:10.1371/journal.pmed.1000332

Li, S., Zhao, J. H., Luan, J., Ekelund, U., Luben, R. N., Khaw, K., . . . Loos, R. J. (2010, August 31). Physical Activity Attenuates the Genetic Predisposition to Obesity in 20,000 Men and Women from EPIC-Norfolk Prospective Population Study. *PLoS Med PLoS Medicine, 7*(8). doi:10.1371/journal.pmed.1000332

Lin, J. (2013, August 28). Fast food: Students struggle with healthy options in short lunch periods. *The Center for Investigative Reporting*. From http://cironline.org/reports/fast-food-students-struggle-healthy-options-short-lunch-periods-5139

Lindsay, K. (2011, February 22). "Weigh Less, Smile More:" How Fitness Magazines Define Health in Very Unhealthy Ways. *Beauty Redefined*. From http://www.beautyredefined.net/weigh-less-smile-more-how-fitness-magazines-define-health-in-very-unhealthy-ways/

Lock, K., Smith, R. D., Dangour, A. D., Keogh-Brown, M., Pigatto, G., Hawkes, C., . . . Chalabi, Z. (2010, November). Health, agricultural, and economic effects of adoption of healthy diet recommendations. *The Lancet*, 376(9753), 1699-1709. doi:10.1016/s0140-6736(10)61352-9

London, B. (2014, January 07). Has 'bikini bridge' become the new thigh gap? Disturbing new selfie fad circulating on social media. *Mail Online*. From http://www.dailymail.co.uk/femail/article-2535098/Is-bikini-bridge-new-thigh-gap-Disturbing-new-selfie-fad-circulating-social-media.html

Lumeng, J. C., Forrest, P., Appugliese, D. P., Kaciroti, N., Corwyn, R. F., & Bradley, R. H. (2010, April). Weight Status as a Predictor of Being Bullied in Third Through Sixth Grades. *Pediatrics, 125*(6). doi:10.1542/peds.2009-0774

Lutz, A. (2013, May 03). Abercrombie & Fitch Refuses To Make Clothes For Large Women. *Business Insider*. From http://www.businessinsider.com/abercrombie-wants-thin-customers-2013-5

Mahoney, J. L., Larson. R. W., Eccles, J. S., & Lord, H. (2005). Organized Activities as Developmental Contexts for Children and Adolescents. In J. L. Mahoney, R. W. Larson, & J. S. Eccles (Eds.). *Organized Activities as Contexts of Development: Extracurricular Activities, After-school and Community Programs* (pp. 4-22). Mahwah, NJ: Erlbaum.

Matt Ryd's Obituary. (2013, August 10). *Chicago Tribune.* From http://www.legacy.com/obituaries/chicagotribune/obituary.aspx?pid=166344182

Maxwell, Z. (2012). Yuck – A 4th Grader's Short Documentary About School Lunch. From http://maxwellproject.com/index.html

Metallinos-Katsaras, E., Must, A., Gorman, K. (2012). A longitudinal study of food insecurity on obesity in preschool children. *Journal of the Academy of Nutrition and Dietetics,* 112, 1949-1958.

Miller, P. E., Reedy, J., Kirkpatrick, S. I., Krebs-Smith, S. M. (2015, January). The United States food supply is not consistent with dietary guidance: evidence from an evaluation using the Healthy Eating Index-2010. *Journal of the Academy of Nutrition and Dietetics,* 115(1), 95-100.

Miller, P. M. (1996, November/December). Redefining success in eating disorders. *Addictive Behaviors, 21*(6), 745-754. doi:10.1016/0306-4603(96)00033-0

Miller, W. R., Rolnick, S. (2002). Motivational Interviewing: Preparing People For Change. New York, NY: The Guilford Press.

Molland, J. (2012, September 14). Why Are Kids Eating School Lunch At 9:45? *Care2.* From http://www.*care2*.com/causes/why-are-kids-eating-school-lunch-at-945.html

Mom Outraged After Athletic Daughter, 11, Receives 'Fat Letter' (2013, October 08). ABC News. From http://abcnews.go.com/blogs/lifestyle/2013/10/mom-outraged-after-athletic-daughter-11-receives-fat-letter/

More U.S. Children Severely Obese, Study Says. (n.d.). *WebMD*. From http://www.webmd.com/children/news/20140407/more-us-children-severely-obese-study-says#1

Morland, K., Wing, S., Roux, A. D., & Poole, C. (2002, January). Neighborhood characteristics associated with the location of food stores and food service places. American Journal of Preventive Medicine, 22(1), 23-29. doi:10.1016/s0749-3797(01)00403-2

Moss, M. (2010, November 06). While Warning About Fat, U.S. Pushes Cheese Sales. *The New York Times*. From http://www.nytimes.com/2010/11/07/us/07fat.html?pagewanted=all

Müller, M. J. (2016, May). Ideal body weight or BMI: so, what's it to be? *American Journal of Clinical Nutrition*, 103(5), 1193-1194.

National Diabetes Fact Sheet, 2011. (2011). *Centers for Disease Control and Prevention.* From https://www.cdc.gov/diabetes/pubs/pdf/ndfs_2011.pdf

Neal, R. W. (2015, January 05). Amazon 'Anticipatory Shipping': New Patent Shows Plans To Ship Products Before Customers Purchase Them. *International Business Times.* From http://www.ibtimes.com/amazon-anticipatory-shipping-new-patent-shows-plans-ship-products-customers-purchase-1545950

Neumark-Sztainer, D., Story, M., & Harris, T. (1999, January). Beliefs and Attitudes about Obesity among Teachers and School Health Care Providers Working with Adolescents. *Journal of Nutrition Education, 31*(1), 3-9. doi:10.1016/s0022-3182(99)70378-x

Neumark-Sztainer, D., Wall, M., Guo, J., Story, M., Haines, J., & Eisenberg, M. (2006, April). Obesity, Disordered Eating, and Eating Disorders in a Longitudinal Study of Adolescents: How Do Dieters Fare 5 Years Later? *Journal of the American Dietetic Association, 106*(4), 559-568. doi:10.1016/j.jada.2006.01.003

Neumark-Sztainer, D., Wall, M., Story, M., & Berg, P. V. (2008, June). Accurate Parental Classification of Overweight Adolescents' Weight Status: Does It Matter? *Pediatrics, 121*(6), 1495-1502. doi:10.1542/peds.2007-2642

New, C. (2012, June 22). Americans Spending Less Money On Groceries, But Greater Share Of It On Processed Food. *Huffington Post.* From http://www.huffingtonpost.com/2012/06/12/american-money-groceries-processed-food_n_1587981.html

Norris, C. (2013, September 6). Chuck Norris says no to school lunch. *WND Diversion.* From http://www.wnd.com/2013/09/chuck-norris-says-no-to-school-lunch/

Ntoumanis, N., Taylor, I. M., & Thøgersen-Ntoumani, C. (2012, January). A longitudinal examination of coach and peer motivational climates in youth sport: Implications for moral attitudes, well-being, and behavioral investment. *Developmental Psychology, 48*(1), 213-223. doi:10.1037/a0024934

Nutrition and Weight Status. (n.d). *Office of Disease Prevention and Health Promotion.* From https://www.healthypeople.gov/2020/topics-objectives/topic/nutrition-and-weight-status

Obesity Alliance Surveys Find Primary Care Practices Not Prepared to Help Patients Manage Weight. (n.d.). *Health Sciences Institute.* From http://www.healthsciences.org/obesity-alliance-surveys-find-primary-care-practices-not-prepared-help-patients-manage-weight

O'brien, K. S., Hunter, J. A., & Banks, M. (2006, May 30). Implicit anti-fat bias in physical educators: Physical attributes, ideology and socialization. *Int J Obes Relat Metab Disord International Journal of Obesity, 31*, 308-314. doi:10.1038/sj.ijo.0803398

Ogden, C. L., Carroll, M. D., Kit, B. K., & Flegal, K. M. (2014). Prevalence of Childhood and Adult Obesity in the United States, 2011–2012. *Survey of Anesthesiology, 58*(4), 206. doi:10.1097/01.sa.0000451505.72517.a5

Olson, C. L. (1994, October 01). Overweight women delay medical care. *Archives of Family Medicine, 3*(10), 888-892. doi:10.1001/archfami.3.10.888

Omli, J., & Wiese-Bjornstal, D. M. (2011). Kids Speak: Preferred Parental Behavior at Youth Sport Events. *Research Quarterly for Exercise and Sport, 82*(4), 702-711. doi:10.5641/027013611x13275192111907

Omli, J., LaVoi, N. M., & Wiese-Bjornstal, D. M. (2008). Towards an Understanding of Parent Spectator Behavior at Youth Sport Events. *The Journal of Youth Sports,* 3(1), 30-33.

Orciari, M. (2012, September 11). Slimming America's waistline: Are we fighting obesity or obese people? *Yale News.* From http://news.yale.edu/2012/09/11/slimming-america-s-waistline-are-we-fighting-obesity-or-obese-people

Overweight and Obesity Statistics. (2013, March 12). *Weight Control Information Network.* From http://win.niddk.nih.gov/statistics/

Park, A. (2011, June 27). Why Being Thin Doesn't Always Mean Being Healthy. *Time.* From http://healthland.*time.*com/2011/06/27/why-being-thin-doesnt-always-mean-being-healthy/

Park, A. (2012, April 18). Tube Feeding: What's Wrong with the Latest Wedding Crash Diet? *Time.* From http://healthland.*time.*com/2012/04/18/with-this-tube-i-thee-shed-whats-wrong-with-the-latest-wedding-crash-diet/

Park, A. (2013, October 10). The Need for Better Obesity Education—In Medical Schools. *Time.* From http://healthland.*time.*com/2013/10/10/the-need-for-better-obesity-education-in-medical-schools/

Pelletier, L. G., Fortier, M. S., Vallerand, R. J. et al. (2001). Associations Among Perceived Autonomy Support, Forms of Self-Regulation, and Persistence: A Prospective Study. *Motivation and Emotion*, 25(4), 279-306. doi:10.1023/A:1014805132406

Persky, S., & Eccleston, C. P. (2011). Medical student bias and care recommendations for an obese versus non-obese virtual patient. *International Journal of Obesity*, 35, 728-735.

Peterman, J. N., Wilde, P. E. (2006). Individual weight change is associated with household food security status. *Journal of Nutrition*, 136(5), 1395-1400.

Physicians Have Less Respect for Obese Patients, Study Suggests. (2009, October 22). *Johns Hopkins Medicine.* From http://www.hopkinsmedicine.org/news/media/releases/physicians_have_less_respect_for_obese_patients_study_suggests

Pollack, A. (2013, June 18). A.M.A. Recognizes Obesity as a Disease. *The New York Times.* From http://www.nytimes.com/2013/06/19/business/ama-recognizes-obesity-as-a-disease.html

Powell, L. M. (2011). Trends in the Nutritional Content of Television Food Advertisements Seen by Children in the United States. *Archives of Pediatrics & Adolescent Medicine, 165*(12), 1078. doi:10.1001/archpediatrics.2011.131

Price, J. H., Desmond, S. M., Krol, R. A., Snyder, F. F., & O'Connell, J. K. (1987). Family practice physicians' beliefs, attitudes, and practices regarding obesity. *Am J Prev Med*, 3, 339-345.

Profiling Food Consumption in America. (2003, March). *Agricultural Fact Book 2001-2002*. From http://www.usda.gov/factbook/2002factbook.pdf

Progress on Childhood Obesity. (2013). *Centers for Disease Control and Prevention.* From http://www.cdc.gov/vitalsigns/ChildhoodObesity/index.html

Puhl, R. M., & Heuer, C. A. (2009, May). The Stigma of Obesity: A Review and Update. *Obesity, 17*(5), 941-964. doi:10.1038/oby.2008.636

Puhl, R. M., & Heuer, C. A. (2010). Obesity Stigma: Important Considerations for Public Health. *American Journal of Public Health, 100*(6), 1019-1028. doi:10.2105/ajph.2009.159491

Puhl, R. M., & Luedicke, J. (2011, September 15). Weight-Based Victimization Among Adolescents in the School Setting: Emotional Reactions and Coping Behaviors. *J Youth Adolescence Journal of Youth and Adolescence, 41*(1), 27-40. doi:10.1007/s10964-011-9713-z

Puhl, R. M., Luedicke, J., & Heuer, C. (2011, October 04). Weight-Based Victimization Toward Overweight Adolescents: Observations and Reactions of Peers. *Journal of School Health, 81*(11), 696-703. doi:10.1111/j.1746-1561.2011.00646.x

Puhl, R. M., Peterson, J. L., & Luedicke, J. (2013, January). Weight-Based Victimization: Bullying Experiences of Weight Loss Treatment-Seeking Youth. *Pediatrics, 131*(1). doi:10.1542/peds.2012-1106

Puhl, R.M., Suh, Y. & Li, X. (2016, April 19). Legislating for weight-based equality: National trends in public support for laws to prohibit weight discriminations. *International Journal of Obesity.* 40:1320-1324. doi:10.1038/ijo. 2016. 49

Rabin, R. C. (2010, March 16). Doctors and Patients, Not Talking About Weight. *The New York Times*. From http://well.blogs.nytimes.com/2010/03/16/doctors-and-patients-not-talking-about-weight/

Rahavi, E., Stoody, E. E., Rihane, C., Casavale, K. O., Olson, R. (2015, February). Updating the dietary guidelines for Americans: status and looking ahead. *Journal of the Academy of Nutrition and Dietetics,* 115(2), 180-182.

Raynor, H.A. & Champagne, C.M. (2016 January 1). Position of the Academy of Nutrition and Dietetics: Interventions for the treatment of overweight and obesity in adults. *Journal of the Academy of Nutrition and Dietetics.* 115: 129-147

Reinboth, M., & Duda, J. L. (2006). Perceived motivational climate, need satisfaction and indices of well-being in team sports: A longitudinal perspective. *Psychology of Sport and Exercise, 7*(3), 269-286. doi:10.1016/j.psychsport.2005.06.002

Richards, A. (2011). Lunch. From http://lunchthefilm.com/

Rideout, V. J., Foehr, U. G., & Roberts, D. F. (2010). Generation M2: media in the lives of 8 to 18 year-olds. *Henry J. Kaiser Family Foundation.*

Robinson, T. N., Matheson, D., Desai, M., Wilson, D. M., Weintraub, D. L., Haskell, W. L., . . . Killen, J. D. (2013, November). Family, community and clinic collaboration to treat overweight and obese children: Stanford GOALS—A randomized controlled trial of a three-year, multi-component, multi-level, multi-setting intervention. *Contemporary Clinical Trials, 36*(2), 421-435. doi:10.1016/j.cct.2013.09.001

Robson, S.M., Couch, S.C., Peugh, J.L.,Glanz, K., Zhou, C., Sallis, J.F., & Saelens, B.E. (2016, April 1). Parent diet quality and energy intake are related to child quality and energy intake. *Journal of the Academy of Nutrition and Dietetcics.* 115: 984-990

Rosenberg, M. B. (2003). *Nonviolent Communication: A Language of Life.* Encinitas, CA: PuddleDancer Press.

Ross, P. (2013, December 30). Vending Machines Must Post Calorie Counts Under Obamacare, Industry Says 'Outrageous' New Regulation Goes Too Far. *International Business Times.* From http://www.ibtimes.com/vending-machines-must-post-calorie-counts-under-obamacare-industry-says-outrageous-1522706

Ryd, M. (2012). Eating Disorder Awareness. From https://www.youtube.com/watch?v=9NU2uJQ_TMA

Samakow, J. (2014, January 30). Teen Starts Petition: 'Make Plus-Size Princesses In Disney Movies!' The *Huffington Post.* From http://www.huffingtonpost.com/2014/01/30/petition-make-plus-size-princesses-in-disney-movies_n_4695664.html

Saper, C. B., Chou, T. C. & Elmquist, J. K. (2002, October 10). The need to feed: homeostatic and hedonic control of eating. Neuron, 36(2), 199-211.

Schlosser, E. (2012). *Fast Food Nation: The Dark Side of the All-American Meal.* New York, NY: First Mariner Books.

Schmidhuber, J., & Traill, W. B. (2006, August). The changing structure of diets in the European Union in relation to healthy eating guidelines. *Public Health Nutrition PHN, 9*(5). doi:10.1079/phn2005844

Schoenfeld, M. A., Tempelmann, C., Martinez, A., Hopf, J. M., Sattler, C., Heinze, H. J., & Hillyard, S. A. (2003, May 05). Dynamics of feature binding during object-selective attention. *Proceedings of the National Academy of Sciences, 100*(20), 11806-11811. doi:10.1073/pnas.1932820100

Schwartz, M. B., Chambliss, H. O., Brownell, K. D., Blair, S. N., & Billington, C. (2003, September). Weight Bias among Health Professionals Specializing in Obesity. *Obesity Research, 11*(9), 1033-1039. doi:10.1038/oby.2003.142

Shewmaker, J. W., & Wardy, M. A. (2011, February 24). Fear of Fat: Preschool Girls and the Thin Ideal. *Pigtail Pals and Ballcap Buddies*. From http://pigtailpalsblog.com/2011/02/fear-of-fat-preschool-girls-and-the-thin-ideal/#. V88-TZMrLBl

Sidani J. E., Shensa, A., Hoffman, B., Hanmer, J., Primack, B. A. (2016, September). The association between social media use and eating concerns among US young adults. *Journal of the Academy of Nutrition and Dietetics,* 116(9), 1465-1472.

Singh, A. (2012, January). Physical Activity and Performance at School. *Archives of Pediatrics & Adolescent Medicine, 166*(1), 49. doi:10.1001/archpediatrics.2011.716

Smith, A. L., Gustafsson, H., & Hassmén, P. (2010). Peer motivational climate and burnout perceptions of adolescent athletes. *Psychology of Sport and Exercise, 11*(6), 453-460. doi:10.1016/j.psychsport.2010.05.007

Spake, A. (2003, June 15). The Science of Slimming. *US News and World Report, p. 38.*

Speers, S. E., Harris, J. L., & Schwartz, M. B. (2011, September). Child and Adolescent Exposure to Food and Beverage Brand Appearances During Prime-Time Television Programming. *American Journal of Preventive Medicine, 41*(3), 291-296. doi:10.1016/j.amepre.2011.04.018

Stanford, F.C. & Kyle, T.K. (2015, December). Why food policy and obesity policy are not synonymous: the need to establish clear obesity policy in the United States. *International Journal of Obesity.* 39:1667-1668; doi:10.1038/ijo.2015.191

Start Smart Development Programs. (n.d.). *National Alliance for Youth Sports.* From https://www.nays.org/programs/start-smart/

Stern, S. (n.d) Managing Opposing Currents: an Interpersonal, Psychoanalytical Technique for the Treatment of Eating Disorders. Chapter 5, p. 86, *Psychodynamic Treatment of Anorexia Nervosa and Bulimia,* edited by Craig Johnson.

Stewart, D. (2012, August 27). Doctor Refuses to Treat Woman Because She's Over 200 Lbs. *Jezebel.* From http://*jezebel*.com/5938169/doctor-refuses-to-treat-woman-because-shes-over-200-lbs

Strong, W. B., Malina, R. M., Blimkie, C. J., Daniels, S. R., Dishman, R. K., Gutin, B., . . . Trudeau, F. (2005). Evidence Based Physical Activity for School-age Youth. *The Journal of Pediatrics, 146*(6), 732-737. doi:10.1016/j.jpeds.2005.01.055

Stunkard, A. J., Sobal, J. (1995). "Psychosocial Consequences of Obesity." In: Brownell, K. D., Fairburn, C. G., eds. *Eating Disorders and Obesity: A Comprehensive Handbook.* New York, NY: Guilford Press, 1995; 417-421.

Styder, D. M., Conviser, J. H., Washburn, J. J., & Aldridge, D. (2014, March). Gender differences in quality of life and functional impairment associated with binge eating disorders: a clinical population study. *International Academy of Eating Disorders.*

Sutin, A. R., & Terracciano, A. (2013, July 24). Perceived Weight Discrimination and Obesity. *PLoS ONE, 8*(7). doi:10.1371/journal.pone.0070048

Swash, R. (2013, November 02). How the 'thigh gap' became the latest pressure point on a woman's self image. *The Guardian.* From https://www.theguardian.com/lifeandstyle/2013/nov/03/thigh-gap-pressure-point-women-self-esteem

Telama, R., Yang, X., Viikari, J., Valimaki, I., Wanne, O., & Raitakari, O. (2005). Physical activity from childhood to adulthood: a 21-year tracking study. *American Journal of Preventative Medicine*, 28(3), 267-273.

TFAH Testifies before Congress on America's Obesity Epidemic during Economic Recession. (n.d.). *Trust for America's Health.* From http://healthyamericans.org/newsroom/releases/?releaseid=164

The Obesity Epidemic and United States Students. CDC. From https://www.cdc.gov/healthyyouth/data/yrbs/pdf/us_obesity_combo.pdf

The School Health Policies and Programs Study. (2006). *Center for Disease Control.*

Thomas, D.M., Ivanescu, A.E., Martin, C.K., Heymsfield, S.B., Marshall, K., Bodrato, V.E., Williamson, D.A., Anton, S.D., Sacks, F.M., Ryan, D., & Bray, G.A. (2014, December 24). Nutritional status, dietary intake, and body composition. *American Journal of Clinical Nutrition.* 101:449-454. doi: 10.3945/acjn. 114. 091520

Thompson, C. (2013, August 28). Some school districts quit healthier lunch program. USA *Today.* From http://www.usatoday.com/story/news/nation/2013/08/27/school-districts-healthy-lunches/2710697/

Thorpe, K. E. (2009, November). The Future Costs of Obesity: National and State Estimates of the Impact of Obesity on Direct Health Care Expenses. *United Health Foundation., The American Public Health Association., Partnership for Prevention.* 1-13. From http://www.fightchronicdisease.org/sites/default/files/docs/CostofObesityReport-FINAL.pdf

Turner, L. R. (2012, February). Student Access to Competitive Foods in Elementary Schools. *Arch Pediatr Adolesc Med Archives of Pediatrics & Adolescent Medicine, 166*(2), 164. doi:10.1001/archpediatrics.2011.837

Unick J.L. Leakey, T., Kent, K., & Wing R.R. (2015, July 14). Examination of whether early weight loss predicts 1-year weight loss among those enrolled in an Internet-based weight lose program. *International Journal of Obesity*. 39:1156-1564; doi:10.1038/ijo.2015.76

Vlahos, J. (2011, April 16). Is Sitting a Lethal Activity? New York Times Magazine. From http://www.nytimes.com/2011/04/17/magazine/mag-17sitting-t.html

Volkow, N. D., Wang, G., Fowler, J. S., & Telang, F. (2008, October 12). Overlapping neuronal circuits in addiction and obesity: Evidence of systems pathology. *Philosophical Transactions of the Royal Society B: Biological Sciences, 363*(1507), 3191-3200. doi:10.1098/rstb.2008.0107

Wake Forest Baptist Study Says Medical Students Under-Focus on Obesity. (2013, October 6). *Winston Salem Journal*.

Wall, M., & Côté, J. (2007). Developmental activities that lead to dropout and investment in sport. *Physical Education & Sport Pedagogy, 12*(1), 77-87. doi:10.1080/17408980601060358

Walsh, B. (2008, June 12). It's Not Just Genetics. *Time*. From http://content.*time*.com/time/magazine/article/0,9171,1813984,00.html

Wardle, J., Haase, A. M., Steptoe, A., Nillapun, M., Jonwutiwes, K., & Bellisie, F. (2004, April). Gender differences in food choice: The contribution of health beliefs and dieting. *Annuals of Behavioral Medicine, 27*(2), 107-116. doi:10.1207/s15324796abm2702_5

Wear, D., Aultman, J. M., Varley, J. D., & Zarconi, J. (2006, May). Making Fun of Patients: Medical Students Perceptions and Use of Derogatory and Cynical Humor in Clinical Settings. *Academic Medicine, 81*(5), 454-462. doi:10.1097/01.acm.0000222277.21200.a1

Weight Loss Options. (2013). *Aspire Bariatrics*. From http://www.aspirebariatrics.com/

Weinstein, A. (2009, August 10). School Lunch Nutrition: What You Need to Know. *Education.com*. From http://www.*education.com*/magazine/article/school-lunch-nutrition/

Weiss, M. R., & Fretwell, S. D. (2005). The Parent-Coach/Child-Athlete Relationship in Youth Sport. *Research Quarterly for Exercise and Sport, 76*(3), 286-305. doi:10.1080/02701367.2005.10599300

Werman, M., & Pillay, K. (2013, September 3). The Secret Behind Finland's Super Smart School Kids? Recess. PRI. From http://www.pri.org/stories/2013-09-03/secret-behind-finlands-super-smart-school-kids-recess

Whitaker, R. C., Wright, J. A., Pepe, M. S., Seidel, K. D., Dietz, W. H. (1997). Predicting obesity in young adulthood from childhood and parental obesity. *New England Journal of Medicine*, 337(13), 869-873.

Whiteman, H. (2013, November 17). Patient-doctor disconnect 'impacts weight loss interventions'. From http://www.medicalnews*today*.com/articles/268872.php

Why we must stop ignoring the psychology of weight loss: Alisa Anokhina at TEDxUCL. (2012, July 02). From https://www.youtube.com/watch?v=NWfqBy4sSD8

Wiersma, L. D. (2000). Risks and Benefits of Youth Sport Specialization: Perspectives and Recommendations. *Pediatric Exercise Science, 12*(1), 13-22. doi:10.1123/pes.12.1.13

Wilfey, & Epstein. (2007).

Wolin, S. J, & Wolin, S. (1993). Bound and Determined: Growing Up Resilient in a Troubled Family. New; Villard Press.

Year two evaluation: Arkansas Act 1220 of 2003 to combat childhood obesity. (2009, May 8). *University of Arkansas for Medical Sciences, College of Public Health.* From www.uams.edu/coph/reports/Act1220Eval.pdf

Young, A., Chaudhry, H. J., Rhyne, J., & Dugan, M. (2010). A Census of Actively Licensed Physicians in the United States, 2010. From http://www.nationalahec.org/pdfs/FSMBPhysicianCensus.pdf

Zimmerman, F. J., & Bell, J. F. (2010, February). Associations of Television Content Type and Obesity in Children. *American Journal of Public Health, 100*(2), 334-340. doi:10.2105/ajph.2008.155119

APPENDIX B
THE *UNWEIGHTED* MODEL OF HEALTH

Characteristics	Dieting	UnWeighted (Early)	UnWeighted (Later)	No Dieting
Weight, BMI, or Numbers:	Primary focus	Some focus	Lifestyle focus	No focus
Rules:	Many	Few	None; only "wants"	None
Restriction:	High	Less	Greater moderation/ greater consistency	No restriction
Deprivation:	Yes	Less	None	Variable
Frequency of Eating:	Determined by diet rules	More frequent	Frequent	Variable
Length of the Process:	3 days to 3 weeks	3 months	Lifetime	Variable
Exercise Intensity:	None or intense	Individually determined	Individually determined	None needed
Exercise Frequency:	Variable	More frequently physically active	More frequently physically active and enjoyed	None
Locus of Control:	External and reward-based	Trend to internal and less external	Greater internal and individual	Unknown
Process or Outcome Focus:	Outcome	Mixed	Process	No process or outcome focus
Self-Talk:	Negative, punitive, and/ or "should" statements	More compassion	Overall accepting and positive	Unknown

Characteristics	Dieting	UnWeighted (Early)	UnWeighted (Later)	No Dieting
Comparing Self With External Standards:	Yes; predominantly external	Less external/ more personal or internal	More internal or personal	Variable
Black or White Thinking:	Yes/all	Less	Little or none	Variable to extreme
Should Statements:	Many	Fewer	Few to none	None
Guilt:	High potential	Less	None	None
Emotional Awareness:	None required	Emerging mindfulness	Substantial	Unknown
Scientific Method:	Not an essential component of most popular diets	Much self-observation and learning encouraged	Ongoing self-observation and learning encouraged	Self-observation and ongoing learning not necessary
Psychological Merit:	None or inconsistent	Some	Substantial	Variable
Scientific Merit:	None or inconsistent	Some	Substantial	Variable
Relationships:	Not specified by the diet	Increased healthy connection	Healthy and sustainable connection	Unknown or variable
Therapist-Counselor Relationship:	Education or diet coaching support encouraged	Counseling or psychotherapy acceptable	Counseling or psychotherapy support acceptable	Role of psychotherapy unknown
Satisfaction:	Short-term effort/long-term promise	Improving short-term and long-term	Substantial short-term and long-term	Often short-term or immediate reward
Success:	Contingent on amount of weight lost	More broadly personally defined	Individually and personally defined	Variable

APPENDIX C
THE ANTI-*BMI* DIET

- Respect and care for the body you have.
- Suspend judgment based on appearance for self and others.
- Engage regularly in physical activities and play that are healthy and enjoyable.
- Eat fruits, vegetables, and healthy proteins that you enjoy frequently.
- Refuse to participate in weight-related competition.
- Endeavor to improve connection in relationships with people and not just relationship with food.
- Use resources in your family and community to support emotional and physical health in an ongoing way.
- Dedicate yourself to being willing to continue to learn about health, wellness, and actualization and to challenge yourself to implement strategies that feel credible and appropriate for you.
- Be active in combating discriminatory attitudes and behavior, especially those related to size-ism and weight-ism.
- Be aware that change is not a perfectly linear path and permit patience and time in all pursuits.
- Permit your own path to success to be uniquely yours and avoid comparing your choices with others.

APPENDIX D
14 WAYS TO ALIGN WITH A PATIENT

- Focus on the patient and their values.
- Be collaborative.
- Enhance the patient's personal goals and perspectives.
- Affirm the patient's right to choose.
- Presume resources for change reside within the patient.
- Be empathic.
- Create an atmosphere conducive to change.
- Be brief in your statements.
- Let the patient fill the space with their talking.
- Withhold judgment.
- Accept that change happens in small steps.
- Recognize seemingly small accomplishments.
- Remember that relapse is a normal part of the change process.
- Be aware that motivation should be considered on a continuum.

APPENDIX E

NUTRITION STRATEGIES FOR PARENTS

❑ Improve nutrient intake:

- Have healthy foods readily available.
- Have prepared meals and snacks ready and available at the appropriate times to avoid over-hunger states.

❑ Improve variety of foods:

- Invite children to try new foods in very small amounts, when possible under non-stressful conditions.
- Introduce new foods to their children, who may otherwise be hesitant to try different foods, by having them see others prepare them, smell them, and eat them.
- Permit and encourage independent likes and dislikes.

❑ Improve frequency of eating:

- Schedule and prepare three meals and two snacks every day.
- Avoid becoming overly hungry.
- Plan for and prepare snacks and drinks that are portable and do not require refrigeration.

❑ Improve the ability of their children to read hunger signals:

- Encourage their attention to degrees of hunger.
- Motivate them to consider what might be satisfying to eat.

❑ Improve the ability of their children to tolerate feelings of fullness or hunger:

- Provide accurate and reliable information about what hunger/fullness signals mean and do not mean.

❑ Reduce the level of ritualistic eating:

- Avoid eating foods in a rigid order.
- Avoid needing to cut foods into a specific number of pieces.

- Avoid rules regarding the number of times a person should chew food items.
- Avoid upset or anger if food routines are unexpectedly changed.

❑ Reduce any urge to engage in competitive eating:

- Avoid all games and contests using food.
- Avoid all games and contests that use drinks of any kind.

❑ Improve their children's independence with regard to food management:

- Provide opportunities to assist with cooking and/or food preparation.
- Try new recipes together.
- Encourage taking turns choosing menu items, as age-appropriate, for the child/adolescent.
- Avoid having any family member be required to eat the same way or required to eat differently than other family members.

❑ Eat in an eating place:

- Avoid eating in front of the television.
- Avoid eating while in the car.
- Create opportunities for eating that permit eating to be a mindful and non-stressful experience.
- Encourage acceptance of others having different eating styles and preferences.
- Avoid being critical of what others are eating.

APPENDIX F
HEALTHY EATING: OBSTACLES & UNDERPINNINGS

❏ *What interferes with healthy eating and why?*

- Lack of variety of foods and flavors
- Hunger
- Insufficient availability of healthy foods
- Difficulty attending to or interpreting hunger cues
- Lack of adequate coping strategies for managing uncomfortable emotion
- Fatigue
- Unavailability of fruits and vegetables
- Sedentary lifestyle
- Comparing body, weight, size, or shape with others
- Value assigned to appearance
- Adopting a thin ideal
- Being critical of one's self or others' weight or shape

❏ *What supports healthy eating?*

- Eating a wide variety of food and flavors
- Opportunities to eat until full
- Food available in plentiful quantities
- Healthy awareness of hunger cues
- Avoiding over-restriction of palatable foods
- Alternative strategies for managing emotion
- Having adequate sleep
- Availability of fresh fruits and vegetables
- Physically active and enjoyable lifestyle
- Respect demonstrated for individuals of all shapes and sizes
- Life satisfaction from relationships, rather than only from food

APPENDIX G

GUIDELINES FOR EXERCISE PROFESSIONALS WITH REGARD TO CREATING A POSITIVE WORKOUT EXPERIENCE

- Truly care about their client's overall well-being.
- Enjoy working with individuals of all sizes.
- Be invested in the client's overall well-being and believe that change is possible.
- Prioritize listening rather than telling.
- Avoid offering nutritional advice or operating outside the limits of their professional license.
- Complete specialty training in working with deconditioned, overweight, and/or specialty populations.
- Prioritize the client's goals, rather than theirs.
- Support the client's focus on goals related to health, vitality, enjoyment, ease of mobility, and other unique personal values.
- Positively reinforce effort and avoid all criticism.
- Avoid lapses to making personal assumptions or judgments.
- Assist clients in being realistic about their personal expectations.
- Avoid using exercise or physical activity as a means of changing shape or weight.
- Be creative in approaching each training moment, but remain safely within the appropriate exercise guidelines.
- Avoid overly strenuous exercise activities, unless discussed with the client and agreed upon.
- Remember that engaging in painful exercise or "going for the burn" may diminish a client's motivation to continue exercise.

- Avoid overreliance, discussion, or over-focus on numbers (weight, Kcals, BMI, etc.).
- Never use numbers to shame or blame.
- Use numbers to guide decisions about exercise prescriptions and training choices.
- Use the numbers to inform personal health awareness and motivate adherence.
- Observe and appreciate the small successes, even if it just involves the client showing up for the workout.

A LIFE OF TRUE SUCCESS

- Living a life that permits being mindful day-to-day of who you are
- Being mindful day-to-day of your physical, emotional, and spiritual health
- Living a life that is both respectful and accepting of yourself and others
- Challenging yourself to set and attain reasonable and meaningful goals
- Attaining balance in your relationship with yourself and others
- Having a life that is oriented to values that you choose
- Finding balance in caring for your personal health and the well-being of others
- Finding compassion and generosity in giving back to your family, friends, and community

About the Authors

Jenny H. Conviser, Psy.D., CEDS, CC-AASP, is a licensed clinical psychologist, Assistant Professor of Psychiatry and Behavioral Sciences in the Feinberg School of Medicine of Northwestern University and a staff member at Northwestern Memorial Hospital in Chicago. Dr. Conviser holds certificates of training in behavioral medicine from the University of Chicago, in Family and Child Psychotherapy from The Family Institute of Northwestern University, and Eating Disorder Certification (CEDS) from the International Association of Eating Disorders Professionals.

Dr. Conviser is regularly consulted for senior professional staff training in esteemed institutions, providing staff training, program development, and intensive care for the most critically ill—life-threatening eating disorders, trauma, co-occurring addictions, mood disorders, and anxiety disorders.

With a master's degree in exercise science, seven years of experience as a NCAA Division I head coach, University of Wisconsin, Madison, and a certification in sport psychology from the Association for Applied Sport Psychology, Dr. Conviser directs sport psychology services at DePaul University and works with athletes, parents, and coaches on achieving peak performance. She also provides sport psychology services for United States Figure Skating's National Champion Silver Medalist (2013), Gold Medalist (2014), and 2014 Sochi Olympics. In addition, Dr. Conviser directs mental training for the United States Figure Skating's senior, elite, and national teams.

Dr. Conviser served as a member of the Advocacy and Communication Committee for the Academy of Eating Disorders (AED), participating in campaigns to reduce weight-related stigma, arguing for reduced use of body mass index measurement in school settings, as well as the healthy weight-related depiction of children in television programming. She has also pioneered research and education in an effort to reduce weight-related stigma in the exercise and fitness arenas.

As a member of the Psychosocial Committee of the Illinois Chapter of the American Academy of Pediatrics, she participates in research, policy development, and physician training for the Pediatric Obesity Prevention Initiative for the development and implementation of a physician/patient communication training programs, which endeavors to improve children's health and well-being throughout the state of Illinois.

Other advocacy projects in which Dr. Conviser is involved include the design, implementation, and analysis of a Northwestern University IRB approved research study, analyzing communication difficulties among bulimic patients who are receiving dental care. The underlying goal of this study was to improve access to dental care for patients who have eating disorders. The results were published in 2013 in the *Journal of the American Dental Association.*

Dr. Conviser is founder and president of Ascend Consultation in Health Care, LLC., which provides clinical behavioral health services in the Midwest and is dedicated to improving access to specialized behavioral medicine services in remote locations. Dr. Conviser enjoys teaching, research, and public speaking on issues related to behavioral health.

Dr. Jason Conviser, Ph.D., FACSM, FMFA, is a fellow of American College of Sports Medicine and fellow of the Medical Fitness Association. He is a leading expert in fitness assessment and exercise prescription for special needs populations. Dr. Conviser is best known for his work with patients dealing with metabolic syndrome, obesity, and providing exercise strategies for those individuals who have "given up." He is the author of eight books targeting fitness related issues. He has also been an invited speaker to 38 healthcare-related international conferences.

In addition, in 2015, Dr. Conviser was featured in the annual volume of *ACSM's Distinguished Leaders Series* DVD, as a professional who has had a noteworthy impact on sports medicine and exercise science. In recent years, he has become a leading expert in the field of bone mineral density and a forceful advocate of osteogenic loading as a modality for addressing bone density issues among older adults.